Aging Well

Other books by James F. Fries, M.D.

Combs, B. J., D. R. Hales, B. K. WIlliams, J. F. Fries, and D. M. Vickery. An Invitation to Health: Your Personal Responsibility. *Menlo Park, Calif.: Benjamin/Cummings Publishing Co., 1983, Revised edition.*

Fries, J. F. Arthritis: A Comprehensive Guide. *Reading, Mass.: Addison-Wesley Publishing Co., 1986, Revised edition.*

Fries, J. F., and G. E. Ehrlich. Prognosis: A Textbook of Medical Prognosis. *Reading, Mass.: Addison-Wesley Publishing Co., 1983.*

Fries, J. F., and L. M. Crapo. Vitality and Aging: Implications of the Rectangular Curve. *San Francisco, Calif.: W. H. Freeman and Co. Publishers, 1981.*

Lorig, K., and J. F. Fries. The Arthritis Helpbook. *Reading, Mass.: Addison-Wesley Publishing Co., 1986, Revised edition.*

Pantell, R., J. F. Fries, and D. M. Vickery. Taking Care of Your Child. *Reading, Mass.: Addison-Wesley Publishing Co., 1984, Revised edition.*

Vickery, D. M., and J. F. Fries. Take Care of Yourself: A Consumer's Guide to Medical Care. *Reading, Mass.: Addison-Wesley Publishing Co., 1986, Third edition.*

Aging Well

A Guide for Successful Seniors

James F. Fries, M.D.

ADDISON-WESLEY PUBLISHING COMPANY, INC.

Reading, Massachusetts ■ Menlo Park, California ■ New York
Don Mills, Ontario ■ Wokingham, England ■ Amsterdam ■ Bonn
Sydney ■ Singapore ■ Tokyo ■ Madrid ■ San Juan

Forms reprinted with permission from *The Power of Attorney Book* by Denis Clifford, published by Nolo Press, 950 Parker Street, Berkeley, CA 94710 (415) 549-1976. Nolo Press publishes a number of books and software on such related areas as estate planning and probate. These include *Nolo's Simple Will Book* by Denis Clifford, *WillMaker* (software/book package available for Macintosh, IBM, Apple, and Commodore) and *For the Record* by Carol Pladsen and Ralph Warner (book/software package for Macintosh). To order copies of any of the above, or to receive a current catalog call toll-free: 800-992-NOLO (US), or 800-445-NOLO (CA, outside 415 area).

Library of Congress Cataloging-in-Publication Data

Fries, James F.
Aging well.

Bibliography: p.
Includes index.
1. Aged—Care and hygiene. 2. Aged—Accidents—Prevention. 3. Aged—Life skills guides. I. Title.
RA777.6.F75 1989 613'.0438 88-35125
ISBN 0-201-51751-5

Cover design: Peter Peckham/Coleman & Christison
Text design: Editorial Design/Joy Dickinson
Production: Michael Bass & Associates
Composition: Composed in 11 point Palatino by The Composing Room of Michigan, Inc., Grand Rapids, Michigan

CDEFGHIJ-DO-943210

Third Printing, November 1990.

Acknowledgments

This book has many roots. In many ways it is the senior sequel to *Take Care of Yourself,* which Dr. Donald Vickery and I wrote in 1975 and have revised many times since. Many of the scientific principles were developed in *Vitality and Aging,* a book written together with Dr. Lawrence Crapo. The work behind the arthritis books, *Arthritis,* and *The Arthritis Helpbook* is further developed here. Experience with large-scale arthritis self-management programs has been very helpful. ARAMIS (American Rheumatism Association Medical Information System), the national arthritis data resource that I direct has provided many insights from our longitudinal studies of human aging. The Healthtrac and Senior Healthtrac programs have inaugurated formal health promotion for seniors, and feedback from some of the many hundreds of thousands of participants has been most helpful. In turn, it is hoped that this book will enrich these programs.

Many people have contributed. I particularly am appreciative of the contributions of Paul Baltes, Ph.D., Margret Baltes, Ph.D., Albert Bandura, Ph.D., Stanley Berney, Walter Bortz, M.D., Gilbert Brim, Ph.D., Lisa Cendejas, Ann Dilworth, Albert C. Fries, Ed.D., Orpha Hair Fries, Sarah Tilton Fries, M. P. H., Harry Harrington, Ed Hemphill, Ph.D., Kate Lorig, Ph.D., Toby Montgomery, J.D., William Patrick, Nancy Richardson, Martin Seligman, Ph.D., John Staples, George Valliant, M.D., Donald Vickery, M.D. Any errors or omissions are my own.

TO OUR READERS

This book is strong medicine. It can be of great help to you. The medical advice is as sound as we can make it, but it will not always work. Like advice from your doctor, it will not always be right for you. This is our problem: If we don't give you direct advice, we can't help you. If we do, we will sometimes be wrong. So here are some qualifications: If you are under the care of a physician and receive advice contrary to this book, follow the physician's advice; the individual characteristics of your problem can then be taken into account. If you have an allergy or a suspected allergy to a recommended medication, check with your doctor, at least by phone. Read medicine label directions carefully; instructions vary from year to year, and you should follow the most recent. And if your problem persists beyond a reasonable period, you should usually see a doctor.

CONTENTS

Foreword

You can age well—with grace and wisdom, wit and experience, energy and vitality. This is realism, not fantasy.

To a considerable extent you can decide whether or not to age. You can choose to age poorly or to age well. But aging well is not easy. It requires some essential knowledge, a good plan, work, and perseverance. You will probably live longer than you think, and you need to plan for it. You need to cultivate a healthy mind in a healthy body, and you will need to find ways to compensate for a slowing biology to achieve your personal potential. You need to avoid major illness. You will be working primarily to improve the quality of your senior years, not to greatly prolong your life. You need to strengthen your mind, your muscles, and your personal relationships. There is no magic formula. There is a successful strategy, but the particular plan and the specific goals must be your own. You need to be in control.

In the opening words of Browning's Rabbi Ben Ezra:

"Grow old along with me
the best is yet to be
the last of life for which the first was made . . ."

How to Use This Book

AGING WELL presents the art and the science behind the manifestations of aging. It can guide you to your own plan for successful aging. This can change your life.

AGING WELL is designed so that each part should be read differently. Part I, "Vitality and Aging," will help you understand the principles of aging well. Part II, "General Concerns," develops the specific practical procedures that you need to implement. Read carefully those sections of particular importance to you. Part III, "Solutions," is for reference. Read this part for help with particular problems that you have now or that develop later. Part IV, "Appendixes," is for background. Read this part to appreciate the meaning of some of the most surprising statistics of aging.

PART I

Vitality and Aging

CHAPTER 1

Aging Versus Vitality

Aging is inevitable. It is that part of the life cycle in which the hair becomes grey, the skin less elastic, the lens of the eye foggy, the reflexes slowed, the risk of disease greatest. Yet it is the time of your greatest wisdom, your richest experience, your deepest insights, your most complete individuality. Successful aging is accomplished by minimizing the physical negatives and optimizing your personal potential.

Consider the implications of these three neglected facts: First, your current life expectancy is probably a good deal longer than you think—you have a considerable period of time to plan for. Second, no matter what you do, you are not likely to change your life expectancy by more than a few months—you will not live forever. Third, you can make dramatic changes in how well you live—you can greatly change the quality of your senior years.

The senior who ages well makes use of the enormous advantages of age. Examples of what can be possible abound in the lives of many vigorous centenarians and seniors in public life. Picasso, Casals, Churchill, de Gaulle, Rubenstein, Basie, Heifitz, and Mao, among many others, demonstrate the potential. Irving Berlin extended his vitality into a second century. George Burns and Bob Hope in their eighties and beyond entertained millions of people. Grandma Moses was still painting at 100. Bertrand Russell was publicly active at 94. George Bernard Shaw was writing at 91. Mary Baker Eddy directed the Christian Science church at 89. Also at 89, Albert Schweitzer headed an African hospital. Michelangelo designed churches at 88. Konrad Adenauer was the chancellor of Germany at 88. Tolstoy took his first bicycle lesson at 67; he celebrated his 70th birthday by riding 20 miles and making love to his wife.

At age 70, Bess James ran 10,000 meters (6.2 miles) in 1 hour, 4 minutes faster than the previous year. Walt Stack at age 73 completed the Iron Man Triathlon with a time of 26 hours and 20 minutes. At age 80 he runs 17 miles a day but complains that he only "shuffles" anymore. Roget continued to update his thesaurus until his death at 90. Elizabeth Arden, founder of the beauty empire, could do a yoga headstand at 75 and was active in the management of her company through age 85. Claude Monet began his Water Lily series at age 76, completing it at age 86. Paul Spangler began training at 67, sedentary and 40 pounds overweight, and set an age record for 10,000 meters (6.2 miles) of 49 minutes 23 seconds at age 80. At age 86 Marshal Tito of Yugoslavia married for the fourth time. At age 88, Frank Lloyd Wright designed the Marin County Civic Center. Leopold Stokowski signed a six-year recording contract at age 94. Tesicki Igarashi climbed Mt. Fugi at 100, having taken up climbing at age 90. When he was 96 and still playing his cello, Pablo Casals commented, "Age is a relative matter. If you continue to work and absorb the beauty of the world around you, you find that age does not necessarily mean getting old."

The potential of the human spirit is clearly long lasting. Some accomplishments, of course, are not possible. Yet the principles that typify those who have aged well are universally applicable. Their achievements are not the achievements of youth. They build on the attributes of age, where long experience, cultivated wisdom, and persistent practice have enabled a wider, more sensible perspective than that allowed to their younger colleagues.

The Bad News: You Can't Live Forever

Human beings are mortal. Like dogs, hamsters, horses, and other animals, we have a fixed average life span. If we do not die of premature illness or accident, we will die a natural death at the end of the natural life span. There are no exceptions to the biological rules that determine the length of life.

The potential human life span appears to average about 85 years of age with an absolute maximum life duration of about 115. The exact genetic limit to life is not very important to personal planning since none of us can estimate our personal life span very accurately and it is different for each of us. For most, it will be between the ages of 70 and 100. Studies of ancient humans suggest that the maximum duration of life has been roughly constant for the past 100,000 years. Intuitively, most of us recognize that eventually the function of our vital organs, which become less efficient with increasing age, will no longer support life, and at this time we will die a natural death of "old age." As disease is prevented by the individual or successfully treated by the doctor, one's "life expectancy" can be increased—a little. Your chances of "premature death" have been decreased. By acting to prevent illness and premature death, you can increase your life expectancy, but not to beyond your maximum biologic life span.

Much past research into human aging has been a quest for the secrets of longevity (and even immortality). Claims that we will soon live to be 200 years old because of massive doses of vitamin C, vitamin E, Gerovital, lifelong jogging, or some other magical device have obscured the more reasonable quest—that for increased vitality in old age.

Errors in the popular press have increased the confusion about longevity. Scientists repeatedly have investigated individuals claiming great age, and in every instance these claims could not be verified. In the United States, the oldest age actually reached has been 114 years. The reasons for exaggerated claims are varied—ignorance, avoidance of military service, attempting to increase prestige, and others—but there is now no question that these claims have been false. Similarly, it has now been proven that there are no secret mountain regions where people live exceptionally long lives.

The "Myth of the Fountain" had its clearest expression in the search of Ponce de León for the legendary Fountain of Youth (thought to be somewhere near the present location of Disney World). The "Fountain" theme is present in the histories of nearly every culture and has its counterpart in rejuvenating elixirs promoted even in our time. Some demographers today have constructed computer models with carefully obscured underlying assumptions to promote similar claims, but this wishful thinking is as misleading as the search for the Fountain.

FIGURE 1.1 *National Survival Curves*

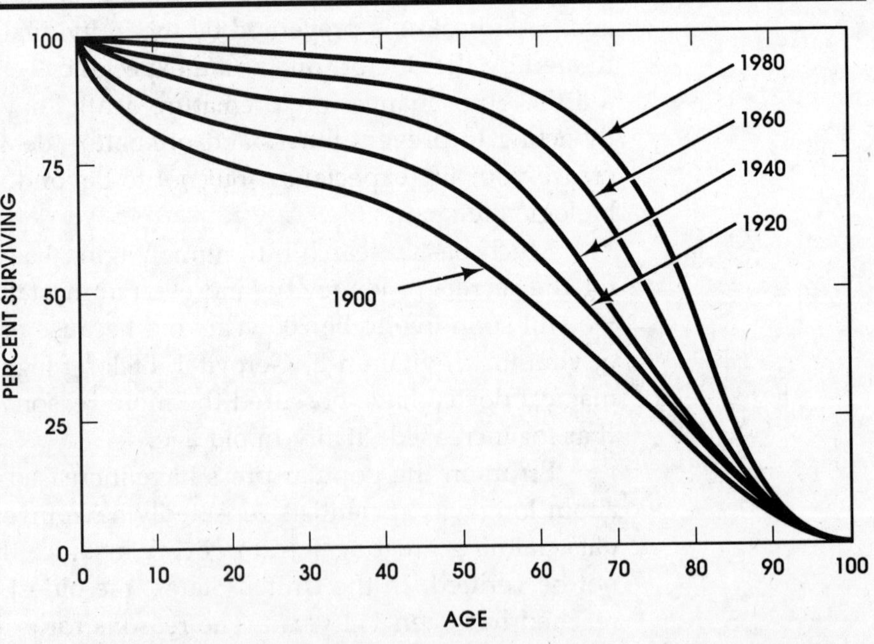

There are indeed ways to slow the aging process, but they have nothing to do with magic fountains or formulas.

Even without magic, however, we can expect to live much longer than could previous generations. The major diseases of previous years, such as smallpox, polio, tuberculosis, dyptheria, tetanus, syphilis, and rheumatic fever, have been nearly eliminated as threats to life. In 1900 the average person died of illness or accident at 47 years of age. Now, the average age of death is nearly 75 years. There are now relatively few deaths in early life. National survival curves, as shown in Figure 1–1, have become more "rectangular" in shape. The end of the natural life span has changed little if at all, as demonstrated by the right-hand "tails" of the curves of Figure 1–1, but life expectancy, on average, is now much greater.

As illness is cured or prevented, it is more common for us to live into "old age"—to live almost to the very end of the natural life span. Obviously, the closer we get to this ideal, the harder it is to make further progress. Barring a breakthrough in life span extension (felt by almost all scientists to be unlikely in the near future), the ultimate human life span will not be greatly changed in our lifetimes. Scientific studies of prevention of disease already have begun to show difficulty in achieving much further reduction of mortality. We must focus our efforts elsewhere. We now must be concerned with the quality of life rather than its duration.

Better News: You Will Probably Live Longer Than You Think

Most of us have been confused by the term "life expectancy." As a result, we expect our lives to be shorter than they actually will be and expect that we (particularly women) will be alone for longer times at the end of life than is likely. After passing the average life expectancies of age 71 for men and 78 for women, many seniors feel that they are living on "borrowed time." Not so.

Table 1–1 demonstrates that the longer you have already lived, the longer your life is likely to be! This is because, having outlived some of your contemporaries, you are now in a better "pool" of longer-lived individuals. Your life expectancy has become better than the average! This is critically important to your life planning; you are very likely to live longer than you might expect if you simply think of life expectancy as 71 for males and 78 for females. At age 70, you have an average of 11 to 15 more years! At age 85, 6 years; at age 100, still over 2 years!

Almost equally important, the differences between male and female life expectancy become smaller with increasing age! While at birth females are expected to live seven years longer than males, by age 70 this gap has narrowed to less than four years, and by age 85 it has narrowed to one year. At age 110 the differences between males and females have entirely disappeared. (Males are subjected to much greater risks of major disease or accident earlier in life; once having survived into their 70s or 80s their life expectancy becomes ever more similar to that of women.) The average differences between men and women are now slowly reducing at all ages. These neglected facts mean that a married couple surviving together into retirement age generally are within a few years of each other in average life expectancy; this should be a major factor in your future planning.

The Best News: You Can Stay Vital

You can slow down your own aging. Almost every important aspect of aging can be modified, by you. The important "age" is not your age in birthdays; it is your biological or "vital" age.

TABLE 1.1. *How Long Do I Have?*

MEN			*WOMEN*		
At Age Achieved	*Additional Years*	*Total Life Expectancy*	*At Age Achieved*	*Additional Years*	*Total Life Expectancy*
65	14.0	79.0	65	18.4	83.4
66	13.4	79.4	66	17.6	83.6
67	12.9	79.9	67	16.9	83.9
68	12.3	80.3	68	16.2	84.2
69	11.8	80.8	69	15.5	84.5
70	11.2	81.2	70	14.8	84.8
71	10.7	81.7	71	14.1	85.1
72	10.2	82.2	72	13.4	85.4
73	9.7	82.7	73	12.8	85.8
74	9.3	83.3	74	12.2	86.2
75	8.8	83.8	75	11.5	86.5
76	8.4	84.4	76	10.9	86.9
77	7.9	84.9	77	10.3	87.3
78	7.5	85.5	78	9.8	87.8
79	7.1	86.1	79	9.2	88.2
80	6.8	86.8	80	8.7	88.7
81	6.4	87.4	81	8.2	89.2
82	6.1	88.1	82	7.7	89.7
83	5.7	88.7	83	7.2	90.2
84	5.4	89.4	84	6.8	90.8
85	5.1	90.1	85	6.3	91.3
86	4.8	90.8	86	5.9	91.9
87	4.5	91.5	87	5.6	92.6
88	4.3	92.3	88	5.2	93.2
89	4.0	93.0	89	4.9	93.9
90	3.8	93.8	90	4.6	94.6
95	2.9	97.9	95	3.3	98.3
100	2.3	102.3	100	2.6	102.6
105	1.9	106.9	105	2.0	107.0
110	1.5	111.5	110	1.5	111.5

SOURCE: 1980 Life Tables, Office of the Actuary, Social Security Administration.

It is how well you function. The differences between your vital (biological) and your actual age can be as much as 30 years.

What is aging anyway? Is it birthdays? White hair? Wrinkled skin? The problem with any definition of aging is that aging is not one thing but many. Scientists have worked with many different "markers" of aging, including blood pressure, skin elasticity, grey hair, cholesterol, reaction time, and lung capacity. None of these markers describes the phenomenon of aging very well, and with each of them some people seem to "age" much more rapidly than others.

In approaching old age, most people fear the loss of the ability to get around easily, loss of intellect and memory, and development of some lingering and painful disease. In sum, people tend to think of old age as dependence on others, inability to take care of themselves, and increasing loneliness and isolation. Old age in this regard has little to do with the number of birthdays, the color of hair, or spots on the skin.

Scientists have now begun to study the differences between individuals, not the averages. Why do some people age more rapidly in particular ways than others? Can we identify the good factors in the "slow agers" and apply them to others? This research is the source of the best news: Many of these factors have been identified, and they can be modified.

Consider the simple paradox of a new exercise program. Scientists note that our ability to run a given distance at maximum speed decreases on average by about one to two percent for every year of life over age 30. This is the result of the aging process; similar declines occur in the reserve function of every body organ. As you grow older, your maximum ability decreases, very slowly.

But beginning exercisers improve steadily even as they grow older. Year after year they can improve their running times and can become physically stronger. Usually it takes five to eight years for a new runner to achieve his or her best running times. Loss of mobility is one of the three great fears of growing old; yet mobility can improve with age, and this can happen regardless of the age at which the exercise activity is started. This potential for increased mobility represents in important ways the ability to reverse the process we think of as growing old.

How can we improve with age when our maximal potential is decreasing slowly each year? The answer: We were not previously functioning at our maximum ability. Few of us are working at our limit in any area; if we are not, then we can improve despite increasing age.

What do we do to improve? The answer is obvious: Practice. If we wish to improve a skill, we must use that skill. If we don't use it, we will lose it. We will rust out, not wear out. If we do not practice a function, that function ages more rapidly.

Can we slow the progression of all aging manifestations? Probably not. At this time it appears that some features of increasing age cannot be altered; some of these are listed in Table 1–2. Most of these features relate to scarring—the accumulation of fibrous scar tissue in our organs. This scarring cannot be reversed, and its accumulation may be one of the causes of the biological limit to our life span.

On the other hand, the listing given in Table 1–3 represents the best news. There are far more aspects of aging that can be modified than cannot, and the most modifiable features are the ones that most of us think of as the most important.

Recent studies have shown that training and practice can improve scores on intelligence tests even in individuals over

TABLE 1.2. *Unalterable Aging Manifestations*

Greying of hair
Loss of skin elasticity
Development of cataracts
Fibrosis and stiffening of arteries
Farsightedness
High-tone hearing loss

the age of 70, that the loss of short-term memory often associated with aging can be improved by practice in related areas, and that reaction times in active people over age 70 can be as quick as those of typical sedentary 20–year-olds. Change has been scientifically demonstrated for each of the important features listed in Table 1–3, which is only a partial list. Most of the crucial aspects of aging, including the presence or absence of disease, are under individual control.

Our society has not encouraged the avoidance of aging, and this has resulted in apparent aging rates that are unnecessarily rapid. We have expected the older individual to be less active, perhaps as a reward for a long period of hard work. We have tried too often to take care of our senior citizens rather than helping our elders take care of themselves. We have not respected the value of accumulated wisdom. We have sometimes required people to retire from activities at an unnecessarily early age. We have failed to recognize that by encouraging disuse we increase financial dependence, remove the individual from the stimulation of new inputs, decrease social

TABLE 1.3. *Modifiable Aging Manifestations*

Features	*Modifying Factors*
Physical fitness	**Exercise, weight control, nonsmoking**
Heart reserve	**Aerobic exercise**
Mobility	**Stretching exercises**
Blood pressure	**Exercise, salt intake, obesity**
Intelligence	**Practice, training**
Memory	**Practice, training**
Reaction time	**Exercise**
Isolation	**Practice, socialization**
Heart disease	**Diet, exercise, other health habits**
Cancer	**Diet, nonsmoking, other health habits**
Arthritis	**Exercise, weight control**
Agility	**Stretching exercises**

interactions that prevent isolation, and reduce the sense of contribution that affects our feelings of self-worth.

A common misconception is that the time for prevention has passed after age 65; that healthy lifestyles undertaken too late in life won't have any effect. In fact, exercise can build cardiovascular strength and reserve to a striking degree at any age. The senior who stops cigarette smoking returns to an average risk of heart attack after only two years and an average risk of lung cancer after ten, and preventive measures can rebuild bone calcium and bone strength in as short a period as one to three years. Actually, healthy lifestyles are *more* important for seniors than for younger individuals, since the risk of disease is so much greater and the positive effects of prevention are realized in a much shorter time period.

Perhaps you see a paradox in that you cannot outlive the life span of our species but that you can modify the rate at which you age. How can this be? The paradox is resolved if we consider the consequences of a nearly unchangeable life span together with a changeable rate for aging. Our vital life can be prolonged, and at the same time our final period of infirmity can be shortened. Dependence and lingering illness can be reduced. Taking care of yourself does not result in a longer old age. To the contrary, what we think of as "old age" is compressed into a shorter period. The period of adult vigor is prolonged.

Psychologists have shown that death is feared less than isolation, infirmity, sickness, depression, and increasing pain in the final days, months, or years. Yet these conditions we fear are the very factors that can be modified and avoided by personal action.

Our society has the same choice that we have as individuals; the central choice is shown in Figure 1–2. We presently have morbidity (illness) concentrated in the later years of life. This illness burden (morbidity) is made up principally of chronic illness, but it also includes the frailties associated with aging. Assuming a future society with an average life expectancy increased to

80 years, one of two possible alternative futures can be imagined. In the first, life expectancy will continue to increase as a result of better medical care and treatment of disease, but the time at which illness or infirmity begins does not change. In this unhappy scenario, the extension scenario, old age becomes fraught with increasing pain, dysfunction, and dependence.

In the second scenario, we have concentrated our efforts on prevention. We have worked to change the age at which

FIGURE 1.2 *Compression or Extension of Morbidity*

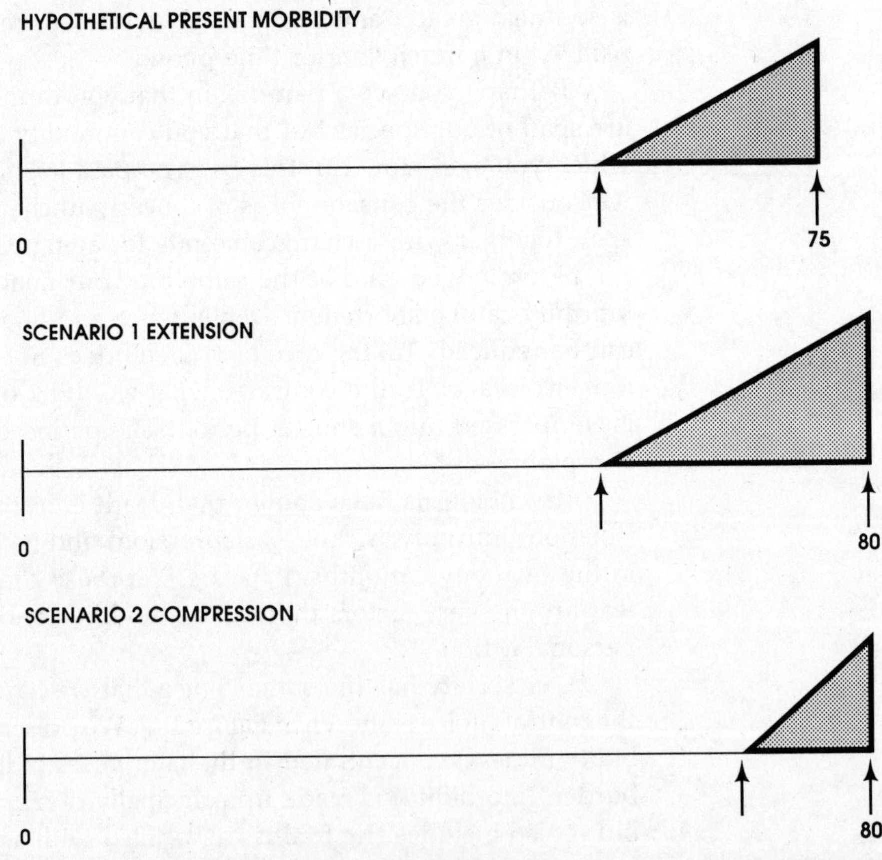

infirmity first becomes manifest. Here, the health problems of the final years are compressed between a later period of onset and the end of life, resulting in *decreasing* problems of illness and senescence. Prevention is *most* important in the senior years. What is possible for the society is also possible for you.

Study of the modifiable aspects of aging has just begun, and it represents a new scientific frontier. Figure 1–3 presents the ideal mortality curves for a society free of illness and accident, which as a society we are approaching. We must begin now to develop similar ideals for our personal health and for our personal function—for the quality of our lives. We are all, as individuals, facing the same frontier.

FIGURE 1.3 *Ideal Mortality Curves*

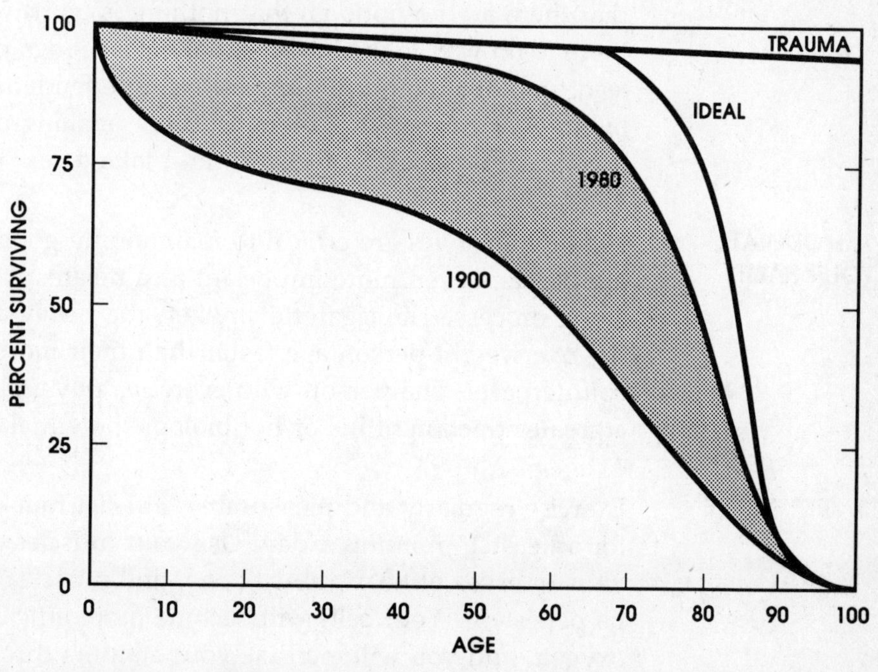

Principal Principles

The principles of aging well are now firmly established. You work to prevent the diseases that make you age faster; you work to avoid the pitfalls. You emphasize expression of your personal choices; you stay in control. You exercise your mind and your body so that the ravages of disuse do not become confused with the aging process.

From the scientific principles outlined above and detailed in the pages to come, the following six basic aging rules become more than platitudes—they describe how to apply the efforts of mind and body to retard aging.

1. MAINTAIN INDEPENDENCE

Independence and confidence are underlying requirements for preservation of vitality. You need to be able to make choices, even small ones, and to thereby alter your future. You need to avoid the situation psychologists call "helplessness," the feeling that there are no options, that nothing is worthwhile and that there is no way to avoid the situation. Feelings of helplessness lead to ill health and to depression. Independence is fostered by emphasizing your personal choices, making detailed plans for the future, looking forward, and taking care of yourself.

2. MODERATE YOUR HABITS

Healthy lifestyles are critical to maintaining good health. They are perhaps even more important as a means of slowing the aging process. The cigarette smoker, the heavy drinker, and the overweight person age faster than their more moderate counterparts. The person who exercises physically achieves a greater fraction of his or her biologic potential.

3. KEEP ACTIVE

Exercise regularly and pleasurably, at least four days a week for at least 15 minutes a day. Use your muscles and build up your reserves of heart, lung, bone, and muscle. Be gentle, but be persistent. Your cells will become more efficient in use of oxygen, and you will increase your stamina through the day.

Stretching exercises will give you flexibility and help you avoid muscle strain. Endurance exercise increases your energy. Walk, jog, bicycle, or swim regularly. Exercise your mind as well as your body. Challenge yourself. Develop the lifelong habit of physical and mental exercise.

4. BE ENTHUSIASTIC

The enthusiasms of youth are tempered by the wisdom of increasing years. Serenity replaces anxiety. This is good. But to stay young you need, in certain senses, to act young. This means that enthusiasm is perfectly permissible. What do you really want to do? Work, travel, sports, hobbies, music, museums? Do it. Plan ahead and savor the anticipation. Look back and enjoy the experience again. Do new things, change hobbies, develop new skills and enjoy them. You are not old as long as you look forward with real anticipation to the future.

5. HAVE PRIDE

Pride is a positive attribute, closely related to what psychologists term "self-image." You must think well of yourself. Individuals with low self-esteem are sick more often, become depressed, and appear to age more rapidly. Pride increases your standards in what you do. It can take almost any form, such as pride in your personal appearance, in home maintenance, in your family, your friends, your work, your hobbies, your play. Be proud of the things that you do well.

6. BE INDIVIDUAL

As you grow older, you are more and more unique. There is no one else with your particular set of life experiences, insights, and beliefs. These are your strengths, and they make you interesting to others. Cultivate this individuality. As you actively grow and change, your personal uniqueness increases. Your individuality is not set early in life but develops as you age. Avoid conformity for its own sake, both conformity with your peer group or conformity with your own earlier behaviors and beliefs. Don't let yourself become perfectly predictable.

CHAPTER 2

Avoiding Possibly Fatal Illnesses

The old adage "an ounce of prevention is far better than a pound of cure" is a sage one. The major health problems of senior America are chronic, long-term illnesses. These illnesses, discussed in this and the following two chapters, make up nearly 90 percent of all the fatalities and about 90 percent of all of the sickness. The good news is that about two-thirds of these illnesses are preventable with present techniques. Even though we think of these diseases as fatal, it is the sickness that they cause more than the fatality that we are trying to prevent.

It is important to understand the basic nature of chronic illnesses such as atherosclerosis, emphysema, osteoarthritis, and even cancer. First, these diseases are universal; we all have them. We differ from each other in how rapidly the tendency toward actual illness is increasing in our bodies. Second, these conditions progress, literally for decades, in a presymptomatic state. You have the tendency toward them, but you don't feel anything bad. The conditions may begin in your 20s, 30s, or 40s and not be detected until perhaps 40 years later. Third, they are slowly progressive unless they are prevented. Fourth, the diseases have "risk factors." Risk factors cause the progression to be more rapid or less rapid than otherwise. Strictly speaking, risk factors do not cause the conditions, but they affect the *rate* of development. The important factor is *how rapidly these conditions are progressing in you.*

Figure 2–1 shows these different patterns of disease development in different individuals. An individual who is developing a condition rapidly may progress to symptoms relatively early, and the condition may even cause death. If the condition progresses more slowly, symptoms are encountered much later in life. If it progresses slowly enough, there may never be any symptoms during the entire life span.

The essence of prevention is to change the rate of development of disease. The goal is to change the rate of unseen progression from the steepest lines of Figure 2–1 toward a less rapid progression.

FIGURE 2.1 *Patterns of Disease Development*

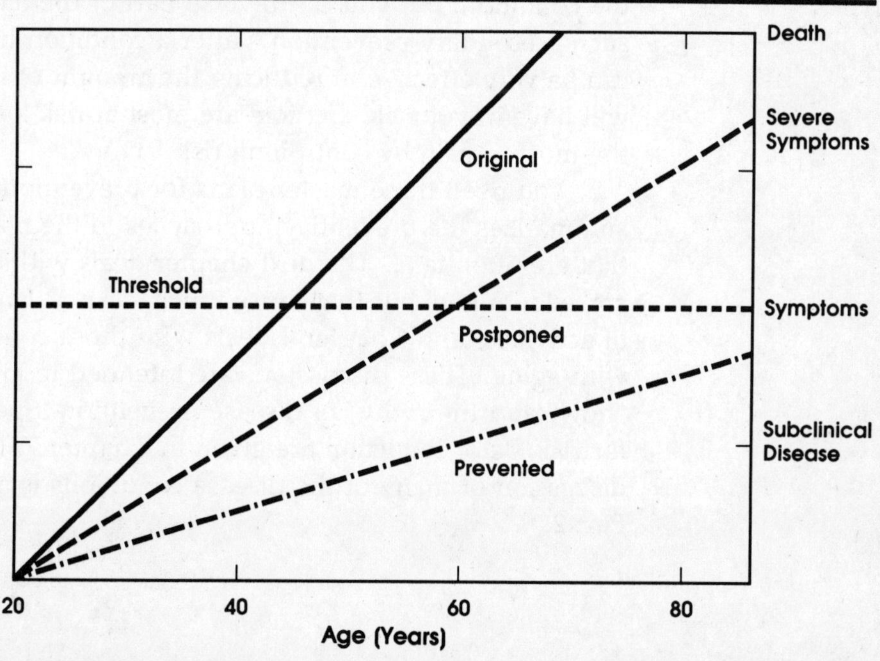

Attention to risk factors is particularly important for seniors. Seniors are approaching or may even have passed the symptom threshold. It becomes critically important to change the rate of progression immediately, before more serious problems arise. Scientific evidence now suggests that prevention will have relatively little effect on the length of life. It will prolong your statistical life expectancy by a small amount, usually only a few months. But what is important is that by practicing prevention you will have major improvement in the quality of your life.

The illness and pain associated with chronic disease are the real problem, and these can be greatly reduced. For example, as mentioned previously, after stopping cigarette smoking you return to normal risk levels for heart attacks after only two years. After ten years you are at nearly normal risk for lung cancer. Exercise programs take only a few weeks to contribute to your health and well-being. For most of the diseases discussed in this chapter, not only can you slow the rate of progression of the condition, but you can reverse part of the damage. Even such "secondary prevention," after a condition has appeared, can be very effective in reducing the amount of illness you will have in your life. Seniors are most at risk and thus have the most to gain by controlling risk factors.

You need three master plans for prevention. This chapter summarizes the preventive approaches to the major diseases that are often fatal. The next chapter deals with diseases that are seldom fatal but that cause much sickness and limitation of activities, and Chapter 4 deals with those conditions associated with aging. These discussions are intended to give you the "how" and the "why" of disease prevention. Specific techniques for risk factor reduction are given in Chapter 7. More detailed discussion of many of the disease conditions is also provided in Part 2.

Prevention of Specific Diseases

Table 2–1 summarizes your master plan for prevention of fatal illnesses. Note that *there are only a few important risk factors that need attention*. The same few risk factors operate to accelerate disease in many categories. Your plan needs to include a good diet, exercise, avoidance of smoking, alcohol moderation, weight control, high blood pressure control, and prudence, exemplified by use of automobile seat belts.

Atherosclerosis

PROCESS Atherosclerosis contributes nearly one-half of the mortality and illness of the senior years. About 40 feet of large and small arteries throughout the body, down to about the size of a soda

TABLE 2.1. *Your Master Plan for Primary Prevention of Fatal Disease*

Disease	*Diet*	*Exercise*	*Avoid Smoking*	*Moderate Alcohol*	*Control Obesity*	*Treat High Blood Pressure*	*Use Seat Belts*
Atherosclerosis	X	X	X		X	X	
Cancer							
LUNG			X				
BREAST	X				X		
COLON	X						
MOUTH			X				
LIVER				X			
ESOPHAGUS			X	X			
Emphysema			X				
Cirrhosis				X			
Diabetes	X	X			X		
Trauma				X			X

straw, are the site of this problem. Small plaques (made mostly of cholesterol) accumulate on the inside walls of the arteries, resulting in narrowing of the arteries. The narrowed and irregular artery now becomes prone to a sudden blood clot (heart attack or stroke). Or, the artery can become so narrow that not enough oxygen-carrying blood can get through (angina, intermittent claudication). The various syndromes depend on the particular artery and whether there is a sudden clot or a continually weak flow. There is now evidence that atherosclerotic plaques that are already in place can shrink in size with diet and, to a lesser extent, exercise. This has been scientifically shown in monkeys and more recently through x-ray dye studies (arteriograms) of human hearts. It is never too late for improvement.

Fatal atherosclerotic events are usually due to heart attack or stroke. These result from sudden formation of a blood clot in the arteries of the heart or brain. There is increasingly good treatment for these clots immediately after they have formed, but not having the clot at all is far better.

Heart attack and *stroke* can also be nonfatal problems involving much pain and disability. Additionally, there are many other nonfatal problems with atherosclerosis. *Angina pectoris* (heart pain) results from inadequate blood supply to the heart muscle, and pain results when exercise or other activities increase the heart's need for oxygen beyond what can be supplied through the narrow artery. *Intermittent claudication* is a similar condition involving the arteries to the legs. Pain in the legs comes during exercise when the leg muscles need more oxygen than they can receive. *Congestive heart failure* results when the heart is unable to pump as much blood as the body needs due to weakening or scarring of the heart muscle. *Transient ischemic attacks* are like little strokes in which momentary clots form in arteries going to the brain. *Multiple infarct dementia* results when recurrent small clots in the brain result in death of brain tissue and thus impairment of thinking and memory. *Impaired kidney function* can result when the arteries leading to the kidney become narrowed.

PREVENTION

Diet is the most important single factor in the prevention of atherosclerosis. The diet should be low in saturated fats, such as those found in eggs, ice cream, butter, and red meat. As a simple rule, these fats are solid at room temperature.

Smoking cigarettes, cigars, or pipes encourages spasm in the walls of the arteries, and avoidance of nicotine can reduce risks of smokers by as much as half.

Control of high blood pressure is important, since the increased blood pressure accelerates the laying down of the atherosclerotic plaques and increases the chances that a weakened artery will blow out. Hypertension is a particularly strong risk factor for stroke. Too much salt holds water in the tissues and increases blood pressure; hence, moderation in salt intake is also important.

Exercise, if it is to help prevent atherosclerosis, needs to be aerobic or endurance in type. That is, it needs to be maintained at least 12 minutes at a session and must be sufficient to raise the pulse rate by 30 to 50 points from resting. This helps teach the heart to become more effective at extracting oxygen from the blood and improves your heart reserve function to protect you if a problem, such as a clot, occurs. Obesity contributes to higher cholesterol levels and decreased physical activity and forces the heart to have to do additional work even at rest.

Cancer

PROCESS

While there are many theories about the development of cancer, in the simplest form you can think of it as *recurrent injury to the cells in a tissue over a long period of time*. The injury causes death of some cells, requires increased cell division, and increases the chance of an error in that cell division so that a malignant cell line is born. With age, the immune surveillance system that usually destroys such malignant cells becomes less effective, allowing the malignant cell line to grow. As the cancer grows, it may directly interfere with local tissues or, commonly, may metastasize and spread to other parts of the body. Cancer accounts for about 20 percent of mortality in the United States. Cancer problems are related to the location of the main tumor but also include pain, weight loss, and problems at distant sites of the body. Complications of radiation treatment, surgery, or chemotherapy add to the illness burden. Prevention is best. Current estimates are that approximately two-thirds of cancers can be prevented with current knowledge!

PREVENTION

Lung Cancer

Approximately 90 percent of lung cancer is caused directly by cigarette smoking. This needless problem is the leading cause of cancer death in both men and women. In men it is now on the decline due to recent trends toward less frequent cigarette use.

Breast Cancer

Breast cancer appears to be importantly influenced by obesity and by high fat diets. The mechanism is not entirely clear, but it appears to involve greater amounts of breast tissue in which to develop cancer and at the same time more difficult detection of an early cancer. Prevention involves weight control and lower saturated fats in the diet. Secondary prevention (early detection) techniques include monthly breast self-examination and yearly mammography, particularly in overweight women with large breasts.

Esophageal Cancer

Cigarette, cigar, and pipe smoking greatly influence risk here, as does heavy alcohol intake.

Mouth and Tongue Cancer

Cigarette smoking, as well as pipe and cigar smoking, accounts for over 90 percent of mouth and throat cancers. The cancers are often, but not always, preceded by development of leukoplakia, whitish patches on the throat or tongue. Smokers should stop; those who don't should regularly inspect the inside of their mouth and throat with a flashlight at perhaps monthly intervals.

Colon Cancer

The dietary factors that influence development of colon cancer have recently become partly recognized. These factors account for about half of these tumors. The key here is enough dietary fiber, such as that found in unrefined grains, fruits, and vegetables. With sufficient fiber, there is less frequent development of precancerous polyps and a greatly decreased likelihood of malignant change.

Cervical Cancer

Cancer of the cervix (mouth of the uterus) has been rapidly declining in women in most developed countries, with the decline perhaps due in part to improved hygiene. The Pap smear is critically important for secondary prevention (early detection) and actually acts in some ways as primary prevention by detecting precancerous changes. For prevention follow your doctor's recommendation for Pap smears; usually this test will be done every two years for senior women.

Cancer of the Uterus

Risk factors are not well established for uterine cancer, but estrogen therapy appears to play at least a small role in some women.

Liver Cancer

Heavy alcohol intake increases manyfold the likelihood of these very difficult-to-treat cancers.

Skin Cancer

The sun is the big culprit with these often minor cancers. Sun exposure, particularly in fair-skinned individuals, causes recurrent tissue irritation, premalignant changes, and then cancer. Secondary prevention is reasonably simple but sometimes neglected. You need to watch your skin for development of new lumps, changes in color of warts or moles, or small sores that don't heal. Cure is almost automatic if you detect and treat these problems early.

Other Cancers No definite risk factors have been identified for cancer of the stomach, the pancreas, the prostate, or the brain, as well as others. Lymphomas and leukemias may result from radiation exposure or from chemotherapy given for other cancers or other diseases.

Emphysema

PROCESS The breathing tubes (bronchi) are kept free of mucus and infection by small hairs (cilia) that move the mucus continually toward the throat, where it is swallowed. Cigarette smoking destroys these cilia so that the mucus cannot be cleared and bacteria can live within the lung. Partial blockage of the breathing tubes make it difficult to exhale, and the inflammation and the increased respiratory effort rupture the small air sacs in the lung, with loss of the surface area necessary for oxygen exchange. This results in slow oxygen starvation, great limitation in function, and usually multiple hospitalizations. The side effects of treatment are often also major problems.

PREVENTION Over 90 percent of emphysema results from cigarette smoking. Pipe and cigar smoking (if not inhaled) does not increase risk. Stopping smoking early in the process will allow stabilization, although this condition does not reverse. Stopping smoking at any point is beneficial.

Cirrhosis

PROCESS Cirrhosis of the liver results from repeated injury to the liver cells, fatty change and death of many of these cells, and accumulation of fibrous scar tissue that ultimately prevents function of the liver. The abdomen may fill up with fluid due to back pressure at the liver; this is called ascites. Jaundice (yellowing) may result from obstruction of small ducts in the liver or from replacement of the normal liver tissue by scar tissue.

PREVENTION

While cirrhosis can follow other kinds of injury, such as hepatitis, over 75 percent of cases are directly caused by long-term heavy alcohol intake, often accompanied by inadequate nutrition. Alcohol intake must be stopped. In early stages, considerable recovery is possible. After heavy scarring has occurred, the condition is not reversible.

Diabetes

PROCESS

As we age, our ability to handle a high sugar load decreases. The glucose stays at higher levels in the blood for longer periods of time. The problem is greatly aggravated by decreased amounts of exercise. As a result, some of this sugar is wastefully excreted in the urine, resulting in the typical early symptoms of frequent thirst and frequent heavy urination. The condition is a relative lack of insulin, since insulin is required for uptake of sugar by the cells. For reasons that are not entirely clear, diabetes itself becomes a risk factor for atherosclerosis and for a set of diabetic complications affecting vision, kidney function, and nervous system function as well.

PREVENTION

Diabetic symptoms beginning for the first time in later life can frequently be reversed completely by simple nonmedical treatment. First, weight loss is important since it decreases caloric need and caloric intake. Exercise is of major importance since it helps the uptake of sugar by the cells from the blood. A diet that emphasizes complex carbohydrates (such as whole wheat grains, cereals, vegetables, and fruits) and that contains adequate fiber is important. This evens out the rate at which the sugars enter the blood so that the body can handle them better.

Trauma

PROCESS

Trauma is not, strictly speaking, a disease, but it results in large numbers of fatalities and even more pain and suffering. Obviously, it is the result of many types of direct injury to the body. Overwhelmingly these injuries, whether to driver, pedestrian, or occupant, are the result of a collision of an automobile.

PREVENTION

Seat belt use is by far the most important single habit to develop to prevent trauma. This is an easy habit, without cost, that reduces risk by over one-half. Remember that seat belt use is for driver and passengers, both in front and back seats. Use of seat belts is a way of achieving greater personal control over your destiny. You think ahead, you plan, and you avoid trouble. It is your choice, far more than you ever imagined, whether or not you stay healthy.

In younger individuals and less frequently in seniors, alcohol or drug intoxication is responsible for many accidents. For seniors, the most frequent danger comes from another intoxicated driver on the road; innocent bystanders are frequently victims.

In the senior years, prescription drugs are a more frequent cause of impairment than alcohol or street drugs. Codeine, Valium, and a whole range of sedatives and tranquilizers can alter the reflexes and the judgement enough to cause accidents. If you have had recent accidents, regardless of whose fault they were, you should seriously consider this possibility in yourself.

Another problem for older individuals has to do with decreased vision, particularly at night. This is common with early problems with cataracts of the lens of the eye or problems with the cornea. Decreased vision at night or seeing halos around lights at night may be the first sign of this potential problem. Don't drive if you are impaired. Don't ride with anyone who is impaired.

The Limits of Prevention

The diseases discussed above are not preventable in all instances. And sometimes you may be suffering from an illness that was caused by something you did early in life, perhaps even at a time when the effects of that action were not well understood. It is important to avoid "victim blaming," or in this instance blaming yourself. The past is past, and you will never know for sure what was the cause of a current problem.

The important principle is that you work for the future. Work for primary prevention of diseases before they appear. Work for early detection and treatment of illnesses that are already there. Even if you already have one or more substantial medical problems, you need to work actively to prevent additional problems in other areas.

Finally, there are a number of major chronic illnesses for which there is no known primary prevention. Some of these are listed in Table 2–2. Some of these eventually may turn out

TABLE 2.2. *Diseases for Which There Is No Known Primary Prevention*

Rheumatoid arthritis	**Ulcerative colitis**
Systemic lupus erythematosus	**Crohn's disease**
Multiple sclerosis	**Parkinson's disease**
Alzheimer's disease	**Polymyalgia rheumatica**

to be infectious diseases or the aftermath of infections. Some may be the result of toxic exposures of as yet unknown type. In some there are hints that risk factors may exist; for example, one study found increased cigarette smoking rates in Alzheimer's disease patients. Even with these diseases there is much that you can do to minimize the distress that they cause.

Improvement of risk factors at any age improves the quality of life. And it does so at essentially no cost (with the exception of medications required to treat high blood pressure). A good diet is of equal or lesser expense than a bad one. Exercise is one of the least expensive uses of your time. Tobacco smoking and alcohol consumption are costly habits. A thin individual has lower food costs than the same individual when obese. Seat belts undoubtedly cost some money, but they are now required by law and are already in all cars.

The major goal of prevention is improvement of the quality of your life in all areas, from vigor and vitality to economic concerns. The quality and pleasure of your life can be materially improved by your careful attention to these few critically important factors.

CHAPTER 3

Avoiding Nonfatal Diseases

More health problems come from "nonfatal" diseases than from fatal ones. Prevention of these problems is critical to your ability to live as well as you can for as long as you can. You probably noticed in the previous chapter that even potentially fatal diseases (like atherosclerosis) cause most of their problems by nonfatal complications such as angina pectoris, nonfatal heart attacks, nonfatal strokes, intermittent claudication, and congestive heart failure.

There are additional disease conditions that are seldom, if ever, fatal but that cause immense amounts of pain and suffering. Osteoarthritis and related syndromes cause nearly one-half of the physical symptoms reported by elder individuals. Little attention has been paid to prevention of these diseases. Yet prevention is possible to nearly the same degree as with the fatal diseases. Secondary prevention of these conditions, after symptoms have begun, is often more difficult. Preventive measures won't always work, but they markedly improve your statistical chances. By working to prevent problems from these conditions, you can strikingly improve symptom levels and the quality of life. Plan ahead, and age well.

Table 3–1 summarizes your master plan for prevention of these problems. Note that again the list of measures required is small, and the list is similar to that required for control of the fatal diseases. The list is led by exercise and weight control, which are essential for preventing these problems as well as others, such as foot problems, not listed. A brief discussion of some common specific problems follows.

Osteoarthritis

PROCESS

Osteoarthritis results from degeneration of the joint cartilage that lines the ends of the bones. As the cartilage becomes weaker, it fragments, and bony and knobby spurs develop at the edges of the joint. The joint becomes stiff and often painful. The syndrome is complicated by subsequent activity limitation and disuse effects.

PREVENTION

Risk factors for osteoarthritis include obesity, inactivity and lack of exercise, and previous injury to the joint. Your preventive strategy is, first, to keep fit. Exercise increases the strength of the bones and the stability of the supporting ligaments and

TABLE 3.1. *Your Master Plan for Primary Prevention of Nonfatal Illness*

Disease	*Exercise*	*Weight Control*	*Avoid Smoking*	*Moderate Alcohol*	*Medication Restraint*	*Diet*
Osteoarthritis	X	X				
Back problems	X	X				
Hernias	X	X	X			
Hemorrhoids	X	X				
Varicose veins	X	X	X			
Thrombophlebitis	X	X	X			
Gallbladder disease		X				X
Ulcers			X	X	X	X

tendons. Exercise nourishes the joint cartilage by bringing nutrients to the cartilage and removing waste products. Regular, gently graded exercise programs are required. Second, control your weight. Being overweight places unnecessary stress on joints by changing the angles at which the ligaments attach to the bone as well as by the additional impact on the feet, ankles, knees, hips, and lower back. Third, protect your joints. Listen to the pain messages that your body sends and perform activities in the least stressful way. Be particularly careful with joints that have sustained injury earlier in your life, since these joints are at greatest risk.

Back Problems

PROCESS

Osteoarthritis also occurs in the joints of the spine and can be aggravated by collapse of spinal vertebrae due to osteoporosis. In younger individuals, problems with herniated intervertebral discs are most common, but by the age of 50 or 60, the disc itself has become more scarred and fibrous and less prone to herniation.

PREVENTION

Exercise is required to keep the muscles that support the back strong. Weight-bearing exercise is important to keep the bone mineral content high and the spinal bones strong. The abdominal muscles must also be strong since they too provide support for the spine. Weight control is the second line of defense; back problems are many times as frequent in overweight individuals. With excess body fat there are unusual and greater stresses, often accompanying lack of exercise, and often reduced muscle strength. Diet is important in that calcium intake should be maintained at substantial levels, with calcium supplements if required, to help keep the bones strong. Previous injury is a fourth risk factor, and, if you have had recurrent back problems, increased attention to exercise and weight control is important.

Hernias

PROCESS

Hernias occur through a combination of weak abdominal muscles and increased pressure within the abdominal cavity resulting from being overweight or from coughing. As a result, small parts of the bowel herniate outward through the inguinal or femoral canals in the general area of the groin.

PREVENTION

Exercise is critical in maintaining the strength of the abdominal muscles. Walking, running, bicycling, and swimming are at least as important as direct exercises to strengthen the abdomen. Weight control helps to improve muscle tone and also to decrease stress. Smoking cessation is extremely important since the chronic smoker's cough more than doubles the risk of these conditions.

Hemorrhoids

PROCESS

This condition, as well as varicose veins and thrombophlebitis, comes from inadequate blood flow in the veins, not the arteries. With hemorrhoids there is slowed flow of blood in the veins around the anus, inflammation, and the development of painful blood clots with surrounding inflammation.

PREVENTION

Exercise programs are important as they keep the body toned and the blood flowing briskly. Sitting a great deal is bad. Overweight contributes to slow flow through the veins through several mechanisms. Local cleanliness around the anus and hot baths act to increase blood flow and reduce inflammation. Perhaps most importantly, straining at stool increases intraabdominal pressure and slows blood flow as well as resulting in local irritation and inflammation as the hard stool passes through the rectum and anus. Singing or talking while on the toilet will help prevent straining—never hold your breath. Take your time, read the newspaper if you need to. Dietary fiber is the natural laxative and is very important. Whole wheat breads and fresh fruits and vegetables are extremely important parts of the diet for this as well as other reasons.

Varicose Veins

PROCESS

Varicose veins result from slow blood flow through the veins of the legs. The veins gradually stretch and become unsightly. Fluid leaking through the capillaries results in swelling of the lower legs and ankles and further aggravates the problems with blood flow. With time, additional veins develop, but these actually aggravate the problem of slow flow.

PREVENTION

Lack of exercise and prolonged standing (without support stockings) are the major culprits. After varicose veins have been present for a while, walking and other exercise is not as helpful as you would like, so early prevention is best. Smoking can contribute in an additional way to development of blood clots. Obesity is a substantial contributing factor in most cases, since the extra weight both requires a larger blood flow and puts pressure on the soft-walled veins, which prevents efficient return of the blood toward the heart. Lose some weight, walk, and use the support hose.

Thrombophlebitis

PROCESS

Here, the stagnation of blood and swelling of the veins in the legs (whether visible as varicose veins or not) results in the development of clots in the leg veins. The blood backs up behind the clot, and then that blood clots also. When the condition is present in large, deep veins, it is hazardous since clots can break loose and travel through the circulation into the lungs where they can cause a condition known as pulmonary embolism.

PREVENTION

The preventive program for thrombophlebitis is identical to that for controlling problems with varicose veins. Exercise helps stimulate the blood flow; obesity makes it worse. Support hose can help. Smoking causes a substantial increase in the likelihood of forming clots. If you have already had one or more episodes of thrombophlebitis, the veins will have sustained damage and the likelihood of recurrence is greater. Blood-thinning medications may be required as part of the secondary preventive process.

Gallbladder Disease

PROCESS

The gallbladder stores the bile salts and cholesterol made in the liver, which are then discharged into the intestine to help in the digestion of fats. These bile salts are soapy substances. They are produced in response to the amount of fat in the diet requiring digestion. Sometimes, these salts can precipitate as stones within the gallbladder itself; the stones often contain substantial amounts of cholesterol. The stones cause local inflammation and if the muscular gallbladder attempts to expel them, blockage of the bile ducts may cause pain, additional inflammation, or jaundice.

PREVENTION

The two risk factors for gallbladder disease increase the likelihood of disease by six to eight times. These are, first, heavy intake of saturated fat and cholesterol in the diet leading to increased bile salt production, and, second, being overweight. Obesity not only greatly increases the frequency of the condition, it makes surgery to correct it more difficult and more hazardous.

Ulcers

PROCESS

Excess stomach acid or other irritants in the stomach or intestine can result in formation of erosions and ulcer craters; often these are large enough to hold a good part of the surgeon's thumb. A breakdown of the protective mucous barrier of the stomach accelerates the damage. We all form small ulcers every now and again, but severe progressive ones lead to pain, major bleeding and hemorrhage, and even perforation all the way through the wall of the stomach or small bowel.

PREVENTION

Stress, in all its forms, is a frequent contributing factor. Smokers have several times more ulcers than nonsmokers, because the constriction of the small vessels prevents adequate nourishment of the wall of the stomach. Negative dietary influences, such as pepper or spices, don't actually play much of a role. Irregular meal habits, by preventing the buffering of the acid by food, often can result in a dietary contribution to the problem. Medications are frequent irritants. Alcohol, particularly hard spirits, can be a culprit. Prescription drugs, such as corticosteroids, aspirin, or other nonsteroidal, antiinflammatory agents such as ibuprofen can also be responsible. Many of the medications that result in ulcers are, in retrospect, found to have been medically unnecessary.

Bladder Infections

PROCESS

If bacteria breed and multiply in the bladder, they cause irritation, inflammation, and painful, frequent, and even bloody urination. The bacteria first have to get there, and this happens most frequently in females since the urethra is short and the bladder not far from the outside. Bacteria usually enter through the urethra. For bacteria to breed, they must be able to multiply more rapidly than they are flushed out of the bladder during the urination process.

PREVENTION

Adequate fluid intake and relatively frequent need for urination is the best prevention. You should drink enough so that your urine is clear, colorless, and copious at least once every day. Hygiene of the genital area is important, since most of the bacteria come from the intestine via the anus. After toilet, women should wipe with toilet paper from front to back so as to avoid transfer of bacteria to the neighborhood of the urethral opening. For early symptoms, drinking cranberry juice in substantial quantities is an excellent secondary preventive. Cranberry juice contains a natural antibiotic that slows the multiplication of the bacteria.

Dental Problems

PROCESS

Bacteria growing within the mouth cavity contribute to plaque, dental decay, and gum disease. The processes and the prevention are well understood.

PREVENTION

Diet is important. In particular, avoid refined sugars and white breads and sugar-containing soft drinks. These are the best food for bacteria. Regular brushing with fluoride toothpaste is important although less so than at younger ages. Dental flossing or use of a rubber tip or toothpicks, on the other hand, is more important and should be performed on a regular basis. Dental checkups are important.

Prevention of Surgery

Not only can the pain and discomfort from the problems discussed in this chapter and from many others be greatly reduced, but you also thereby have a good chance of avoiding the need for a variety of types of surgical operations. Thus, without a hernia you don't need a surgical hernia repair. Surgery for hemorrhoids isn't ever required if you don't have hemorrhoids. You can decrease the likelihood of gallbladder surgery. You can decrease the requirement for gastric resection or other complex procedures for treating ulcers. You can decrease the likelihood of needing coronary artery bypass surgery. Surgical operations are expensive, uncomfortable, and always involve some degree of risk. Reducing the need for such treatment is a major bonus.

The popular press always emphasizes the fatal problems. To age well, it is even more important to prevent the common chronic illnesses that give you a lot of trouble over a long time period.

CHAPTER 4

Avoiding Some of the Problems of Aging

Some of the problems that occur as we age are part of the aging process itself. They result from the stiffening and scarring in our tissues that increase as we get older. They result in a relative frailty of our entire bodies and of particular body parts. Here too, you are in control. To a great degree, you can slow down the aging process.

The line between problems of chronic disease and problems of aging is a very blurred one. For example, arthritis has some aspects of an aging process and some of a specific disease. In our arteries, the accumulation of fats on the inside of the arteries, called atherosclerosis, is generally felt to be a disease. On the other hand, arteriosclerosis, the stiffening of the walls of the arteries together with loss of elasticity in the artery walls appears more likely to be an intrinsic part of the aging process. Further, many problems such as memory loss or medication side effects are general concerns of aging. These are not diseases either, but they cause many difficulties.

The problems discussed here are discussed later in Part 2 in more detail, but some of the points bear repeating. This chapter emphasizes, by use of some examples, that there *are* solutions to problems of aging just as with problems of disease, that these solutions require advance planning, and that your plan can yield concrete positive results.

Table 4–1 summarizes your master plan for prevention of some frequent problems of aging. The diet you need includes sufficient calcium (see Chapter 7) in addition to the factors that we have discussed earlier of low fat, high fiber, and low salt. The exercise that you need to undertake should be not only physical but also mental, as you jog the memory and strengthen the mind. The checkups, which are important for early detection and appropriate treatment of some of these problems, need to be done both by yourself and, in some instances, by health professionals.

Osteoporosis

PROCESS

As we age, we gradually lose calcium from our bones. The bones become less strong, more brittle, and thus more prone to fracture. This process is called osteoporosis. It occurs particularly rapidly in women after the menopause, since estrogen seems to be important in maintaining bone strength. About 650,000 fractures occur each year in the United States as a result of osteoporosis.

TABLE 4.1. *Your Master Plan for Prevention of General Problems of Aging*

	Diet	*Exercise*	*Checkups*
Osteoporosis	X	X	
Falls and fractures	X	X	
Medication side effects			X
Cataracts			X
Corneal opacification			X
Hearing loss			X
Memory loss		X	
Dependence	X	X	X

PREVENTION

Exercise (and estrogen supplementation in women) is required for strong bones. Exercise must be weight-bearing so that it stresses the bones and gives a signal to the body to lay down more calcium and strengthen the bones. Walking, jogging, and even standing provide such stress. Strengthening the bones of the spine is particularly important since this is the site of over half of the osteoporotic fractures.

Calcium is as important as exercise, but in a secondary sense. Without exercise, the calcium is not used by the body, so no matter how much calcium you take in, you don't get an effect. You need the signal from the bones to the metabolic systems of the body that more calcium is needed; then the calcium is absorbed by the small intestine, transported to the appropriate part of the body, and laid down as new, strong bone. Your last two years of exercise are most important; within two years, people who stop exercising lose the benefits. On the other hand, sufficient exercise can maintain bone strength at the normal levels of younger life for an indefinite period. A new exercise program can substantially strengthen weak bones.

Falls and Fractures

PROCESS

Falls cause an astonishing amount of difficulty for older individuals. Falls may result from frailty, slowed reaction time, lack of conditioning, poor vision, poor hearing, presence of medical disease, or a whole variety of different problems that are common in older people. The key is to think of the impact as well as the fall. (It isn't the falling that is the problem; it is hitting the ground.) This means that you have to think about your environment as well as about your physical condition.

PREVENTION

Certainly you want strong bones; the approach to preventing osteoporosis has been outlined above. You want your body to be as strong as possible, and this entails all of the principles described throughout this book. Then, you need to consider the dangers in your environment. Loose throw rugs, absence of good lighting, failure to use nonskid tape in the bathtub, absence of hand rails in difficult places, and other such factors are very important. What about your vision? Think through a typical day, imagine those places where it is most likely that you might fall, and make a plan to reduce the danger. Go through the same process for each person with whom you live—if they break something, it will decrease the quality of your life.

Medication Side Effects

PROCESS

As we age, we are subject to more side effects from lesser amounts of drugs. This is because the body mechanisms that eliminate drugs from our system are less effective, and our liver and kidneys do not work as quickly to excrete these substances from the body. Drug side effects become extremely common, and *most of them are not even recognized*. Instead, the side effects are thought of as problems in their own right. Common drugs like codeine can cause depression and sleepiness. Simple tranquilizers like Valium can muddy your thinking and your memory. Aspirin becomes more irritating to your stomach even though you may not feel the early symptoms as keenly. *Somewhere between 10 and 20 percent of hospital admissions for seniors are the direct result of medication side effects*. Most of the medications that cause the side effects are not medically required.

PREVENTION

This potential problem needs constant attention. We tend gradually to accumulate an overflowing medicine chest. New drugs are started more frequently than older ones are discontinued. Usually your entire medication program is seldom reviewed at the same time, either by you or by your doctor.

There is only one sure way to avoid medication side effects and that is to take no medications at all. At the most basic level, you should always ask yourself whether elimination of all medicines might be possible. If you think this might be feasible, then talk it over with your doctor. At the least, you and your doctor may develop a plan that involves many fewer medications, even if they cannot all be eliminated.

You can stop over-the-counter drugs by yourself. Ask yourself if you really need the medication. Try for a while without it and see if any problems come up. Talk over any questions with your doctor. Repeat this process at least every six months, and prune your medications back to those that are truly important.

Cataracts

PROCESS

The lens of the eye focuses the light for our retina and allows us to see well. As we age, the lens begins to accumulate scar tissue, so that eventually, in many persons, light does not penetrate through the lens as it should. Decreased vision, particularly at night, comes first. Ultimately, blindness can result. The same process is generally going on in both eyes, although often at quite different rates.

PREVENTION

We don't know any way to prevent the scarring in the lens, but the medical problem of loss of vision can be very effectively treated. Cataracts are treated by cataract surgery. A surprising number of people do not notice the slow decrease in vision with cataracts and delay the corrective operations far too long. This results in needless decline in the quality of life. Be alert for loss of vision. Cover one eye and then the other and check to see if vision is equal. Be particularly alert for problems with depth perception or in seeing at twilight or after dark. Have a formal eye examination yearly, and more often if you seem to be having problems.

Corneal Opacification

PROCESS

The cornea is the outer covering of the eye and is also a lens. The same things happen to it that happen to the lens, although usually later, and often less seriously. The process of the cornea becoming opaque can result in blindness.

PREVENTION

There is no direct way to prevent corneal opacification. Fortunately, it is less common than cataracts. As with cataracts, you need to be alert for changes in vision, and you need to call these to the attention of a health professional. Corneal transplants and special types of contact lenses are effective in countering this problem. The usual mistake is to wait too long for correction, thus decreasing the quality of life in the interval.

Hearing Loss

PROCESS

The delicate hearing apparatus in the middle ear (and the ear drum itself) becomes stiffer with age, causing gradual loss of hearing in almost all individuals, with loss of high-tone hearing occurring before loss of lower-tone hearing. Loss of hearing obviously makes communication more difficult. Equally importantly, hearing loss decreases the inputs that you need to make your memory and your thinking work well. Many problems that are written off as "senility" turn out to be only problems with hearing loss.

PREVENTION

There is no known way to prevent the occurrence of hearing loss (although once in a while the problem is only wax buildup in the ear canals). However, hearing aids and devices that will restore hearing to essentially normal levels are readily available. Your task is to be sensitive to any loss of hearing and to take up the corrective measures early. Otherwise, a whole series of unnecessary problems of communication and apparent loss of intellect can result, and the quality of your life will be less than it should be.

Memory Loss

PROCESS

With age, the speed of transmission of impulses through our nerves slows. Our brains contain ever larger amounts of material to remember. We tend to lose the ability to concentrate as closely on new facts, names, and events. Many of the items in our memory store will not have been remembered recently and thus will be in inactive parts of the brain for retrieval. The sum of all these things results in loss of memory, particularly for recent events, and this is unfortunately usually ascribed just to "age". Memory lapses then become frightening occurrences, resulting in fear that we are losing our minds and becoming senile.

PREVENTION

The underlying physical processes of memory loss are not preventable, but most of the manifestations are. Correcting hearing, using lists to compensate, concentrating on new information by using specific techniques, and a variety of other approaches discussed in detail in Chapter 10 can help. You need to exercise your memory.

Dependence

PROCESS

Avoiding dependence is one of the central themes of this book. To the extent that your body does not work well, you may unnecessarily require help from others. To the extent that your mind does not work as well as it should, you may also require outside help. If you contract a specific illness or disease, preexisting dependence may make you more susceptible to debilitation than necessary.

PREVENTION

Prevention of dependence begins with a state of mind. Independence needs to be a primary goal. Then with the help of this book you can work backward to protect the abilities that protect your independence. You need to believe that you can remain indefinitely independent, in the most important senses of the word. Then you need to commit yourself to a plan, and then to execute it. More on this later.

Using Your Master Plan for a Better Life

Avoiding and compensating for the declines of aging are in large part possible by use of your master plan. The independent senior life is the end of a chain of events, and you control most of the events in the chain. You want to seek optimal physical health and optimal mental health, and thus achieve the life of your own choice that is the essence of successful aging.

CHAPTER 5

Avoiding the Stereotype

Successful aging requires breaking the conventional stereotype of the old person. This stereotype is widely held by the nonsenior population and, unfortunately, is tacitly accepted by many seniors. The stereotype is summarized in Table 5–1; you can avoid it, and this is part of aging well.

Consider the very negative impact of this false stereotype. The older individual is seen as slow and enfeebled and often in the way of younger vigorous individuals. These problems are seen as aggravated by a frequent discourtesy, either in holding up a queue without regard to the people behind or ignoring the long line of cars crawling behind. The older individual is seen as incapable of productive action or behavior.

Mentally, this conventional stereotype centers around rigidity and inflexibility. The older individual is seen as self-centered, opinionated, and not open to new information. Stereotypically, the older individual repeats himself or herself frequently, whether it is the same old stories, the same proverbs, or a rigid, stereotyped response to the same general question even though the situation may have changed. The older person is seen as frequently more interested in the trivial than the more important, and may argue over pennies or be extremely concerned over the smallest part of a large issue.

Socially, the old stereotype of aging centers around the older person as a drain on other resources, whether these be public monies or family time. The older person is to be listened to politely because of old debts, but remarks and opinions do not need to be taken as of consequence. The burgeoning number of older individuals is seen as constituting a major economic threat to the health of the nation that will increase markedly over future years and that will require construction of many more hospitals and nursing homes. Stereotypically, all old people are seen as about the same—to be tolerated, to be given a pseudorespect that is not really meant, and, essentially, to be ignored. The productive days of the older person are seen as past, and social interactions are only helping them mark time to death.

TABLE 5.1. *The Old Stereotypes of Age*

PHYSICAL	
Feeble	**Drives slowly and discourteously**
Slow	**Causes accidents in others**
Gets in the way	**Nonproductive**
MENTAL	
Crotchety, irascible	**Repeats the same old stories**
Opinionated, impossible, rigid	**Not really interested in young people**
Not open to new ideas	**Overly critical of other generations**
Argues over small sums of money	**Lives in the past**
SOCIAL	
Needs to be patronized	**Uses up family resources**
Eats at the public trough	**Requires pseudodeference**
Uses up hospital beds	**Poses an increasing economic threat**
All old people are about the same	**Aged individuals are only marking time to death**

Facing the Stereotype

You need to understand this stereotype of older people and its consequences. You should personally evaluate which, if any, of the many facets apply to your own actions and activities. This kind of introspection can guide you to areas of potential change that can open up your life and improve your relationships. Remember that a stereotype is nothing more than an easy way to classify people that is narrow in scope and in most cases just plain wrong.

Pay particular attention to the seldom-discussed issue of perceived discourtesy. This is one of the easiest areas to change, and your actions here contribute positively toward relations between the generations. For example, studies indicate that one of the major differences between older drivers and younger ones is failure of seniors to use the rearview mirror. This failure can contribute directly to automotive hazards (particularly with rear-end or turning accidents), but it also makes it impossible to notice that a number of cars are trailing and that their drivers are fuming. Thus if you pull off the road at a safe and convenient place, everyone else can proceed more comfortably toward their destination. Similarly, although you don't want to give up your right to completely understand a purchase price or complicated form, you can use your greater time flexibility to plan your day so as to select times and places at which you can get complete and unhurried attention without affecting others.

Creating a New Stereotype

Age must not be considered as a long list of negative traits without easy solutions. The older citizen usually is productive and able. Paul Newman, Katherine Hepburn, Henry Fonda, and Jimmy Stewart, among many others, exemplify a mature grace and excitement. The positive attributes far outweigh the negative; yet they are strangely unrepresented in the traditional stereotype. It is time for a new stereotype.

The new characterization of aging probably shouldn't be termed a stereotype at all. Older individuals are more different, one from the other, than are younger individuals. Lifetimes of widely differing experiences create uniqueness, not conformity.

Many of the specific advantages of age are listed in Table 5–2. Physically, the older individual is active. Where limitations are present, they are compensated for in a variety of ways. Actions are deliberate, carefully chosen, and effective. The increased amount of time for discretionary use is an immense positive attribute and can be used to achieve objectives not possible for individuals more strictly tied to job and family. Your local environment can be kept bright and clean and your contributions rich and unusual.

Mentally, the central value of age is wisdom. Wisdom results from a huge backdrop of accumulated memories and experiences that bring unique perspectives to new problems.

TABLE 5.2. *The New Characterization of Age*

PHYSICAL	
Active	**Is deliberate and effective**
Compensates for limitation	**Uses time positively**
Contributes in unusual ways	**Is sensitive to courtesy issues**
MENTAL	
Wisdom and counsel	**Has huge store of accumulated memories**
Learns actively	**Has unique perspectives and experiences**
Seeks new inputs	**Seeks new experiences**
SOCIAL	
Relative affluence	**Volunteers constructive efforts**
Rich network of good friends	**Looks forward and plans**
Empathetic and helpful	**Seeks and enjoys activities**

Wisdom consists of the application of experience to a new situation similar in some ways to old situations frequently faced but additionally with novel elements. Thus wisdom requires not just experience but detailed appreciation of the nuances of the immediate situation. The activated elder seeks new information and experiences so as to apply the experience of the past to the problem of the present.

Socially, seniors are also extremely different, one from the other. As a class, much can be made of the relative affluence of the older population. Seniors on average have more money than any age group except 45- to 64-year-olds, and in general they have fewer obligations to family and others. Of course, this characterization can be overly optimistic when applied to the situation of some individual seniors; many seniors are below the poverty line. Also, senior assets are often present in the form of house and land equity and are relatively difficult to convert into active income. Many seniors are on low, fixed incomes and are especially vulnerable to the problems of inflation. Nevertheless, the positive aspects of senior finance seldom receive enough attention. Seniors represent an immense market for new goods and services and provide economic power and capital to a growing national economy. When all elements are considered, seniors are *not* a drain on national resources. Seniors pay a large fraction of property and sales taxes as well as income taxes. They endow, to a large degree, our universities and our symphonies. Seniors are central to our economy.

Moreover, the senior has a rich social network of good friends, with shared experiences going back over many decades. With relative freedom of time, seniors contribute the lion's share of volunteer efforts to society. Altruism, an attribute everyone wants, is increasingly feasible for the senior freed from some of the competitive pressures of time and work. The increased freedom in choosing which activities to pursue and how to spend each day contributes to personal satisfaction. The ability to learn in new areas and to undertake new directions is increased rather than diminished.

The new characterization of age, therefore, should be seen in essence as flexibility, not rigidity. Aging provides an opportunity, with greater freedom from constraints of tight schedules and heavy personal obligations. More choice is possible, and there are more options to exercise. Aging in many ways represents freedom.

CHAPTER 6

The Psychology of Healthy Aging: Choices, Coping, Optimization, and Growth

Much has been made of the dependence of seniors. Indeed, this is a central feature of the old, pessimistic stereotype of aging discussed in the preceding chapter. Psychologists and gerontologists, on the other hand, have emphasized that the central feature of healthy aging is *independence*. These two concepts, increasing dependence and increasing independence, seem to contradict one another. However, they are not true opposites. You do not need to give up independence merely because you are more dependent. Independence and dependence can coexist, and often it is necessary that they do so.

Dependence means, essentially, that you need the help of others. You cannot do everything yourself. It is an accepted fact that no one can be completely self-sustaining anymore. We are *all* dependent on others. Most of us do not grow our own food, cut our own hair, build our own shelters, or repair our own automobiles. Our complex service society allows individuals to specialize at things they do well and to choose to be dependent on others in other areas. If we are more affluent, we may choose to have people mow our lawns, wash our cars, clean our houses, and cook meals for us at home or at restaurants. We never *could* do all things for ourselves. We were always dependent.

If an older individual requires or desires additional help in meal preparation, household management, or physical

TABLE 6.1. *Psychological Structures for Better Health*

Avoid Learned Helplessness
Action: Consider setbacks as accidental, isolated events that will be over soon.
Develop Self-Efficacy
Action: Recognize that your choices can change your future, and exercise your right to choose.
Choose the Right Coping Strategies
Action: With personal crises, work to see a good side to them, and cope by using humor and altruism.
Optimize Selectively and Compensate
Action: Choose your favored areas for growth and use whatever aids you need to achieve your goals.
Use the Life Cycle to Your Advantage
Action: Use the positive attributes of age to achieve the goals of age.

assistance, this is just a slight change in degree from the dependence that we have practiced and enjoyed all our lives. It is part of making our living more efficient.

Independence has to do with being able to make the choices, not to perform all the actions. You have to be able to direct, in small ways or large, your future. Aging well does not require ability and competence in all areas. It requires the ability to plan and choose.

Psychologists have developed these simple principles into a number of formal theories of aging. Five major psychological contributions are discussed here. They are summarized in Table 6–1. These theories are not mutually contradictory. Rather, they complement each other, each illuminating particular problem areas and appropriate actions to counter the problem.

Avoid Learned Helplessness

Dr. Martin Seligman, Professor of Psychology at the University of Pennsylvania, has developed and experimentally tested the theory of "learned helplessness." Helpless behavior is learned in a vicious cycle in which continued failure leads to setbacks that lead to a failure to even try to succeed that, in turn, leads to further setbacks. Animals placed in hopeless situations gradually learn that effort is futile and that escape is impossible. They become sad, inactive, and resigned. Humans in analogous situations, such as with chronic illness, often gradually change their behavior in the same negative ways. Efforts are not initially rewarded, a feeling of helplessness is learned, and the individual drifts into depression, inactivity, and poor health. This theory can be considered a metaphor for some societies, in which an absence of opportunity gradually conditions a society into despondency and despair.

The brighter side of the learned helplessness theory is that not everybody is susceptible to this vicious cycle. The key to avoiding learned helplessness is what is termed "explanatory style." Suppose that you drop a plate and it breaks. There are two alternative ways that you can explain this event to yourself. One person may say, in effect: "I am clumsy, I am always dropping and breaking everything, I have always been this way, I am clumsy in everything that I do." This is the explanatory style that leads to learned helplessness. The reason for a problem is attributed to a personal fault and that fault is seen as long lasting and extending to everything that the individual does. With this explanatory style every adverse event in life becomes additional evidence that life is helpless and hopeless. Depression and poor health result.

With the same event, another individual may say, in effect: "Plates break, it just happened, I'll sweep it up and throw out the pieces, it doesn't affect anything else in my life." This explanatory style sees the event as just an accident, of short duration, which only affects the one small area of life. This better explanation of the same event does not promote the vicious cycle of learned helpless behavior. It is generally much closer to the reality of the event. It leads to good continued psychological and physical health.

Develop Self-Efficacy

Dr. Albert Bandura, Professor of Psychology at Stanford University, has developed the concept of "self-efficacy." Self-efficacy means that you believe that you can exercise some control over events in your life. The term "self-efficacy" refers to people's belief in their capabilities. Effective functioning requires not only skills but the self-belief to use them well.

People who believe that they can produce changes have better physical and psychological health than people who believe that nothing they do matters. Obviously, if you believe that your choices can have an effect, you are more likely to engage in activities and to maintain the effort needed to succeed. If you believe that you can stay healthy and vital by your own choice, then you *can* stay healthy and vital. The positive results from your actions create a cycle of positive reinforcement that contrasts with the negative vicious cycle that can result in self-discouragement.

Dr. Kate Lorig, Dr. Halsted Holman, and I have developed a self-management program for patients with arthritis. In this course, patients are taught (and teach themselves) hundreds of ways to help control the problems of their arthritis through exercise, relaxation, pain management techniques, and a variety of other approaches. Individuals going through this course (now offered nationally through the Arthritis Foundation) have been shown in many separate experiments to do much better than people who don't take the course. For many people the course plays a larger role in helping them with their arthritis than does their medication.

We carefully studied the many thousands of people in these arthritis self-management courses to find out just which parts of the program were the most effective. Here, there was a surprise. All the different elements of the course helped, but the major factor, which correlated most strongly with the decreased pain and increased function experienced by participants, was not the specific tips and tricks, but instead the increase in self-efficacy that resulted from the course! Patients began to recognize that their own actions could make a difference and that they could improve. And they did.

Choose the Right Coping Strategies

Dr. George Valliant, Professor of Psychiatry at Dartmouth University, has looked at the strategies that individuals use in coping with major life problems. He has carefully studied the lives of a certain group of men over many decades. Many major problems arose in the lives of these men: divorce, death of spouse, illness, job loss, and others. It was the way in which the men coped with the crises rather than the occurrence of the crises that predicted their future health.

There are many ways of coping with crises. You can deny that the event ever happened, get angry, be bitter, drink heavily, or distort the facts of what happened. All these are likely to result in subsequent poor health. On the other hand, there are "mature" coping mechanisms. Those individuals who worked to see the best in a bad situation, who anticipated better events later, and who coped by using humor and altruism were those who subsequently experienced good health. You can laugh at your foibles and a good many of your health problems, you can minimize them to yourself, or you can use them as a stimulus to help others. When you do so, the problems grow less and may even disappear.

Optimize Selectively and Compensate

Dr. Paul Baltes, Professor of Psychology at the Max Planck Institute in Berlin, and Dr. Margret Baltes, Professor of Psychological Gerontology at the Free University of Berlin, have introduced the concept of "selective optimization with compensation."

This is a complex but very important concept in which the words "selective," "optimization," and "compensation" are all important.

The concept derives from two central observations made repeatedly by specialists in aging problems. First, things do become harder to do with age. It takes longer to improve a skill, and it takes more effort in order to improve. Second, it has been abundantly proved that performance in many important human activities can be improved, despite age, at almost any age. Thus, people can become physically stronger, can learn to improve their memories, can improve performance on intelligence tests, and can improve skills at many different activities even when the activity is newly taken up late in life.

The paradox, observed by the Drs. Baltes and coworkers, is that while growth and improvement in nearly all functions are theoretically possible, in practice there is not enough time in the day to improve them all given that it takes more time and effort to improve as we grow older. Thus, we must seek to optimize abilities in areas of particular importance to us to facilitate lifelong growth, and at the same time we must be *selective* in choosing those areas we wish particularly to work on.

Moreover, our approach toward *optimization* of a particular function need not proceed in the same manner that it might have when we were younger. We may have to compensate. We may choose an adjacent or different goal because resources, physical strength, or handicap might decrease the chances of success with a particular strategy. The positive attributes of age, as discussed in Chapter 5, are employed wherever possible. It is said that there are many ways to skin a cat (although I don't personally know anyone who has even tried one way). If one solution doesn't work, try another. *Compensation* implies that we need to take a careful look at our strengths and abilities and choose the most effective techniques for us.

An interesting corollary of this theory is that *we must give up in order to gain*. In order to gain enough time to grow in desired areas, we must give up activities in other areas.

The accumulation of essentially trivial habits and activities is one of the secret problems of aging. The very number of these little things adds up to keeping us from having the time for something new. This is the principle behind sabbaticals for university professors. By freeing time from routine rituals, time is created for new interests and activities.

The same opportunity is present for seniors. What can be simplified? What can be given up with profit? Depending on the circumstances, you might gain from not reading the second and third newspaper or any of the six magazines, by resigning from two clubs and three committees, by choosing to live with a friend or by deciding it is time to live alone. Television time (game shows and police dramas) is an obvious source of new time for you. Shopping expeditions can be rationed, and the frequency of laundry and house cleaning might decrease. Some people gain freedom by selling the car, others by moving to smaller dwellings with greater services. The little daily habits are like garages or attics; they become gradually cluttered with things of little consequence, and they need to be periodically cleared out.

Use the Life Cycle to Your Advantage

Dr. Gilbert Brim, author and member of the MacArthur Foundation's Committee on Successful Aging, has spoken and written widely about the "life cycle," as have others. A few years ago there was a tendency for scientists to view life as a period of growth in the early years, followed by a period of plateau, followed by a period of slow, gradual decline. This concept was in many ways responsible for the negative stereotype of aging.

In contrast, life cycle theorists see various stages to the life cycle, each one with its own advantages and disadvantages. Childhood, adolescence, early adult life, and maturity all have their problems, challenges, and pains, each offset by their particular pleasures and opportunities.

Optimal maturity requires that the positive attributes of the mature part of the life cycle be applied to the solution of its problems. Grace, serenity, time, experience, and wisdom are powerful attributes. With age, issues can be approached in greater depth, considered more deliberately, and choices executed on the basis of a more varied and richer experience.

Even more importantly, there is time to think about the meaning of things. Dr. Brim recommends an autobiographical effort as a way to approach a deeper understanding of your own life, its relations to others, and its current strengths. Your personal autobiography is not intended to challenge the best-seller list. It is a serious effort for you to perform a life review, to go systematically year by year through your past, to remember, and to write out those major events and many minor ones that make up your life. It needs to have both the good and the bad, the problems and the solutions. It has no one format; it can emphasize events or friends, problems or experiences. It can be a treasure for children and grandchildren. Research into family genealogy can have similar benefits and can help transfer wisdom between the generations. Nearly everyone who undertakes a systematic life review is immensely rewarded by the experience. There is just so much there. And so much of it has been nearly forgotten and displaced from consciousness.

Growth

Independence depends on the number of choices you elect to make for yourself. Making plans, anticipating, and executing choices are the keys to independent living. By so doing you improve your efforts, avoid learned helplessness, improve your belief in your own self-efficacy, become prepared to cope with the inevitable crises, and are able to grow and develop in those areas that you choose throughout your life cycle.

Exercising choice does not mean that you need to look around for large decisions to make. Small ones are just as important. Among nursing home residents those who *choose* to do something as simple as taking care of a potted plant or who choose when to see a movie have been proved to receive substantial improvements in health and satisfaction. It is not the small action itself that creates the benefit; rather, it is the resulting sense of personal control that improves health and well-being. Exercising choice does not mean that your choices have to be something that others will approve. Often the mature part of the life cycle is the time to be a bit of a nut.

I know a number of very successful senior lives that have centered around a single activity taken up late in life. One person became an accomplished bird watcher, another a connoisseur of vintage automobiles. Several that I know joined a 50+ runners club and have pursued goals of physical fitness to an extreme; some have volunteered to work toward control of Parkinson's disease, and others to get out the vote for their political party. One walked the Pacific Coast trail by himself. One tutored English to underprivileged youngsters and another became a skilled and respected docent for a local botanical park.

In these very brief discussions of complex psychological theories, I have avoided discussion of the plentiful scientific evidence behind the various concepts and have undoubtedly, by oversimplification, not done justice to theories developed by my friends and colleagues. I have tried to indicate, however, that from these many different viewpoints, scientists have developed a realistic optimism about the possibility of more optimal maturities. The several lessons help to provide a framework within which to develop your personal plans.

PART II

General Concerns

CHAPTER 7

Five Keys to a Healthy Senior Lifestyle

Seniors benefit more than anybody else from good health habits. You have a higher likelihood of encountering the problems that result from poor health habits over a shorter period of time. A small change in your health risks provides greater benefit to you than does a large change in a younger individual. It is never too late. The last two to ten years of your health habits are the critical ones. The improved physical function afforded by good health habits is increasingly important to the quality of your life. Good health habits improve your ability to do well when you encounter accident or illness.

Good news—there are only five major areas: exercise, diet, smoking cessation, alcohol moderation, and weight control. Actually, for most individuals, *you don't even need to worry about five areas, but fewer yet*. Probably you are already a nonsmoker. Probably your body weight is not too far from where it needs to be. Probably your alcohol intake is already moderate. Probably you already do some exercise, and probably you already have some good dietary practices. Make your own personal inventory of what needs attention. It may well be quite a short list. Make your choices, make your plan, and get on with it.

Exercise

Exercise is the central ingredient of good health. It tones the muscles, strengthens the bones, makes the heart and lungs work better, and helps prevent constipation. It increases physical reserve and vitality. The increased reserve function helps you deal with crises. Exercise eases depression, aids sleep, and aids in every activity of daily life.

THE THREE TYPES OF EXERCISE

There are stretching exercises, strengthening exercises, and aerobic or endurance exercises. You need to know the difference between the three types.

Strengthening exercises are the least important, and you can do them or not. These are the "body building" exercises that are often performed just for cosmetic results. They build more bulky muscles. Squeezing balls, lifting weights, and doing pushups or pullups are examples of strengthening exercises. These exercises can be very helpful in improving function in a particular body part after surgery (for example, knee surgery) where it is necessary to build back strength. Otherwise, do them only if you like to.

Stretching exercises are designed to keep you loose. These are a bit more important, and everyone should do some of them, but they don't have many direct effects on health. As you age, you want to be careful not to overdo these exercises. Toe-touching exercises, for example, should be done gently. Do not bounce. Stretching should be done relatively slowly, to the point of early discomfort and just a little bit beyond.

Stretching exercises can be therapeutic in certain situations. If you have a joint that is stiff because of arthritis or injury, if you have just had surgery on a joint, or if you have a disease condition that results in stiffness, then stretching is usually an important part of the therapeutic solution. Remember that there is nothing mysterious about the stretching process. Any body part that you cannot move through its full normal range of motion needs to be repeatedly stretched so that you slowly, often over weeks or months, regain full motion of that part.

For most people, however, stretching exercises are useful mainly as a warm-up for aerobic or endurance exercise activity. Gently stretching before you begin endurance exercise can begin to warm up the muscles, make them looser, and decrease the chances of injury. Stretching afterward can help prevent stiffness.

Aerobic (endurance) exercise is the key to fitness. This is the most important kind of exercise. The word "aerobic" means that during the exercise period, the oxygen (air) you breathe in balances the oxygen you use up during the exercise period. During aerobic exercise, a number of body mechanisms come into play. Your heart speeds up in order to pump larger amounts of blood. You breathe more frequently and more deeply to increase the oxygen transfer from the lungs to the blood. Your body develops increased heat and compensates by sweating to keep your temperature normal. You build endurance.

During endurance exercise periods, the cells of the body develop the ability to extract a larger amount of oxygen from the blood to increase function at the cellular level. As you become more fit, these effects persist. The heart becomes larger and stronger and can pump more blood with each stroke. The cells can take up oxygen more readily. As a result, your heart rate when you are resting doesn't need to be as rapid, allowing more time for the heart to repair itself between beats.

AEROBIC EXERCISE

Aerobic exercise is important at all ages. You are never too old to begin an aerobic exercise program and to experience the often dramatic benefits. There are, of course, a few differences in beginning an exercise program later in life. If you have been deconditioned by avoiding exercise for some time, you are likely to start at a lower level of physical ability than would a younger person. You may be more susceptible to fractures if you fall and injure yourself. You may have an underlying medical condition that limits your choice of exercise activities. You may need to talk with your doctor for advice as to exactly how to proceed. Nevertheless, at your age you need aerobic exercise more than ever, and there is almost always a way to achieve it.

Some people worry that exercise will increase their heart rates and that they have only so many heart beats in a lifetime and they may be using them up. In fact, because of the decrease in resting heart rate, the fit individual uses 10 to 25 percent fewer heartbeats in the course of a day, even after allowing for the increase during exercise periods. Aerobic training also builds good muscle tone, improves reflexes, improves balance, burns fat, and makes the bones stronger.

Much has been made of reaching a particular heart rate during exercise that avoids too much stress and yet provides the "training effect." Cardiologists often suggest that a desirable exercise heart rate is 220 minus your age times 75 percent. Table 7–1 lists these target values depending on your age. Usually it is difficult to count your pulse while you are exercising, but you can check it by counting the pulse in your wrist for 15 seconds immediately after you stop exercising, and then multiplying by 4. More importantly, as your training progresses, you may wish to count your resting pulse, perhaps in bed in the morning before you get up. The goal here (if you do not have an underlying heart problem and are not taking a medication such as propranolol that decreases the heart rate) is a resting heart rate of about 60 beats per minute. An individual who is not fit will typically have a resting heart rate of 75 or so.

TABLE 7.1. *Target Heart Rates During Exercise*

Age	*Beats Per Minute*
60	120
65	116
70	112
75	109
80	105
85+	101

We generally find this whole heart rate business a bit of a bother and somewhat artificial. There really are no good medical data to justify particular target heart rates. You may wish to check your pulse rate a few times just to get a feel for what is happening, but it doesn't have to be something you watch extremely carefully.

There are easier ways of telling how you are doing. Endurance activity is a bit uncomfortable at first and then becomes quite comfortable as your training program persists. It is not "all out." You should be able to carry on a conversation while you are exercising. On the other hand, you should be breaking a sweat during each exercise period if the exercise is performed at normal temperatures of approximately 70 degrees (except swimming, of course). The sweating indicates that the exercise has raised your internal body temperature.

Aerobic exercise must be sustained activity. You need at least 10 or 12 minutes of exercise each session. You can progress up to 200 minutes per week, spread out over five to seven sessions; beyond this amount no further benefit seems to result.

Your choice of a particular aerobic activity depends on your own desires and your present level of fitness. The activity should be one that can be graded. That is, you should be able to easily and gradually increase the effort and the duration of the exercise.

Walking by itself is not always an aerobic exercise, but it provides very important health benefits. If you haven't been exercising at all, start by walking. For seniors, a gradual increase in walking activity, up to a minimum of 200 minutes per week, usually should precede attempting a more strenuous aerobic program. Walking briskly can be aerobic, but you need to push the pace quite a bit to break a sweat and get your heart rate up a bit. Walking uphill or upstairs can quite quickly become aerobic.

Jogging, swimming, and brisk walking are appropriate for all ages, and many seniors of all ages participate. Masters swim programs are increasingly popular. Inside the house, stationary bicycles or cross-country ski machines are good. We have seen people confined to bed using a specially designed stationary bicycle. Some individuals like to use radio earphones while they exercise; others exercise indoors while watching the evening news. While almost any activity from gardening to tennis can be aerobic for some, remember that the exercise can't be start and stop. Aerobic activity can't come in bursts; it must be sustained for at least a 10- to 12-minute period.

CAUTIONS ABOUT AEROBIC EXERCISE

If you have a serious underlying illness, particularly one involving the heart or the joints, you may want to ask your doctor for specific advice. Advice from your physician should always take precedence over recommendations in this book. For most people, however, the doctor's advice is not required. We recommend mentioning your exercise program to your doctor while on a routine visit for some other cause. A good doctor will encourage your exercise program and perhaps guide you in choosing goals and activities.

Some doctors will recommend that you have an electrocardiogram or an exercise electrocardiogram before you start exercising. It is difficult to see what this accomplishes, since gentle graded exercise is a treatment for heart problems anyway, but the test does little harm. Many doctors don't think that these tests are necessary, regardless of age, unless there are specific known problems. If a doctor recommends a coronary arteriogram before you begin an exercise program, you should seek a second opinion to see if this somewhat hazardous test is needed.

"Crash" exercise programs are always contraindicated. You have to start gently and go slowly. There is never a hurry, and there is some slight hazard in pushing yourself too far too fast. Age alone is *not* a contraindication. Many seniors who have achieved record levels of fitness as exemplified by world class marathon times have started exercising only in their 60s, 70s, or even 80s. As mentioned earlier, Mount Fuji has been climbed by a man over 100 years of age.

GETTING STARTED

Assess your present level of activity. This is where you start from. Set goals for the level of fitness you want to achieve. Your final goal should be at least one year away. You may want to develop more proximate goals for what you would like to achieve at one, three, and six months. Select the aerobic activity you want to pursue. Choose a time of day for your exercise. Develop exercise as a routine part of your day. We like to see exercise regularly performed, every day, for at least five out of seven days of the week. If you exercise all seven days, take it easy one or two days each week. Younger individuals can frequently condition with exercise periods three times a week, but for seniors more gentle activities performed daily are more beneficial and less likely to result in injury, particularly when you are getting started. You can make ordinary activities like walking or mowing the lawn "aerobic" by doing them at a faster and constant pace.

Start slowly and gently. Your total activity should not increase by more than 10 percent each week, and exercise each day should be no more than 10 percent or so above that of the typical exercise day. Each exercise period should be reasonably constant in effort. If you are walking, jogging, or whatever, you can use both distance and time to keep track of your progression. When starting out, it is a good idea to keep a brief diary of what you do each day to be sure you're on track. It is generally best to first slowly increase your weekly exercise time to a total of at least 90 or 100 minutes before you work to increase the effort level of the exercise. Get accustomed to the activity first, and then begin to push it just a little bit. Again, progress slowly.

Be sure to loosen up before and after exercise periods and to wear sufficiently warm clothing so as to keep the muscles from getting cold and cramping. The bottom line is patience and common sense.

HANDLING SETBACKS

No exercise program ever goes smoothly. After all, you are asking your body to do something it hasn't done for a while. It will complain every now and again. Even after you have a well-established exercise program, there will be interruptions. You may be ill, take a vacation where it is difficult to exercise, or sustain an injury. Most people starting exercise programs have two or three minor injuries in the first year and thereafter have problems less frequently. Sprained ankles, tendonitis, falls, and even dog bites are common. These are frequent setbacks, but they shouldn't change your plan. Common sense is the key to handling setbacks. Often you can substitute another activity for the one you are having trouble with and thus maintain your fitness program. Sometimes you cannot, and you just have to lay off for a while. When you start back again, don't try to start immediately at your previous level of activity; deconditioning is a surprisingly rapid process. On the other hand, you don't have to start at the beginning again. The general rule is to take as long to get back to your previous level of activity as you were out. If you cannot exercise for two weeks, gradually increase activity over a two-week period to get back to your previous level.

TOPPING OUT

After your exercise program is well established, you need to make sure that it has become a habit that you want to continue for a long time. As indicated, there is no medical evidence that more than 200 minutes a week of aerobic exercise is of additional value. This is about half an hour a day. Many people will not want to exercise this much, and that is perfectly fine. You can get most of the benefits with considerably less activity. At 100 minutes a week, you get almost 90 percent of the gain that you get with 200 minutes. At 60 minutes a week, a total of 1 hour, you get about 75 percent of the benefit that you get with 200 minutes. After you have a well-established exercise program, dropping the frequency back to three or four times a week is all right, and will maintain fitness.

Exercise should be fun. Often it doesn't seem so at first, but after your exercise habits are well developed, you will wonder how you ever got along without them. Once you are fit, you can take advantage of your body's increased reserve to vary your activity a good bit more than you did during the early months. You can change exercise activities or alternate hard and easy exercise days. At this point we hope you will be a convert to exercise programs. You can work to introduce others to the same benefits.

Diet and Nutrition

A variety of dietary considerations are important to the healthy life. The main factors are summarized in Table 7–2. In general, you should move slowly in making changes from your present diet. Most people don't like sudden, radical changes in their diet. As a result, if they try, they may give up the changes after a while. Instead, you should move gradually toward improvement. Good dietary habits exist over a continuum; you don't have to change them all at once. The farther you go, the greater the benefits.

FAT INTAKE

Excessive dietary saturated fat is the worst food habit—greasy kid stuff! Saturated fat intake is the major cause of atherosclerosis (including heart attacks and strokes). Cholesterol checks are OK for motivation, but dietary changes should be made by everyone, regardless of their cholesterol level, since everyone will benefit. A good cholesterol goal is 175 or less. Native Japanese on traditional diets average a cholesterol of under 100! Important new evidence suggests that atherosclerotic plaques that have already built up on the inside of your arteries can decrease in size and, in some instances, nearly disappear with sufficient dietary change. This has been shown both in monkeys given high-fat (atherogenic) diets and in arteriographic studies of human hearts.

Cholesterol levels are only a very rough guide to your dietary needs. The actual chemistry of fats in the body is very complicated. The waxy white cholesterol not only comes in your diet; it is also manufactured by your liver. This production in turn is related to the various other fats in your diet. Attached to the cholesterol itself are high-density lipoproteins (HDL), which help prevent atherosclerosis, and low-density lipoproteins (LDL), which make serious problems much more likely. The LDL travels "outbound" from the liver and can deposit on the inside of vessel walls. The HDL takes cholesterol "inbound" back to the liver for excretion and can help remove plaque from arterial walls. Many laboratories measure serum cholesterol quite inaccurately. Hence we are not too enthusiastic about using

Table 7.2. *Your Diet for Health*

Protein

Slightly decrease total protein. Increase protein from whole wheat grains, vegetables, poultry, and fish.

Fat and Cholesterol

Decrease total fat intake to less than 30% of total calories. Greatly decrease the saturated fats of whole milk, most cheeses, eggs, red meat. Switch to vegetable oils, soybean oil, corn oil, peanut oil, olive oil.

Carbohydrate

Increase total carbohydrates emphasizing whole wheat grains, vegetables, cereals, fruit, pasta, rice.

Alcohol

Moderate use or less; "moderate" approximates two drinks daily.

Fiber

Increase fiber intake with emphasis on fresh vegetables and whole wheat grains.

Salt

Decrease to about 4 grams per day from present average intake of 12 grams a day. Avoid added salt in cooking or at the table and heavily salted foods. Further decrease if medically recommended.

Caffeine

Limit to 300 mg a day or less, equivalent to three cups of coffee.

Calcium

At least 1,000 mg per day for men, 1,500 mg per day for women. Nonfat milk has 250 mg per glass. Use powdered nonfat milk in things like soup. If necessary, consider supplementation with calcium carbonate (Tums, Oscal).

serum cholesterol levels as the sole measures of your own dietary needs. Everyone will benefit from further decreasing fat intake. You cannot have too low a cholesterol level.

You can simplify this whole complicated business simply by cutting down on the *largest* sources of the bad fats in your diet; compensate by slightly increasing the good fats. The worst fatty foods are butter, whole milk, eggs, and animal fats. Fortunately, there are approaches to changing intake of these major foods that are pretty easy to take. With *eggs* you just have to cut down the number per week; two eggs a week is a good ultimate ration. For *butter*, use margarine instead. The best margarines are the softest ones. For *milk*, just use lowfat or nonfat. The calcium and other nutrients in milk are very good for you. For *animal fats*, decrease the frequency of red meat. A good rule for many people is to avoid having red meat two days in a row. This is an easy rule, and it gets variety into your diet. When you do have red meat, choose a less tender cut, trim the fat extensively before cooking, broil so that the fat burns or runs off during cooking, and cook the meat a little more well done. (Outside barbecuing should probably be limited to 30 times or less each year since theoretically there are some carcinogens in the charred meat; for most people this isn't a restriction.) Don't fry foods; this adds fat. Watch out also for palm oil and coconut oil; although vegetable oils, these are also saturated fats and bad for your arteries.

What to increase in your diet? *Fish* is excellent, and you should plan for at least two fish meals a week. Interestingly, the best fish for you are the high-fat fishes that live in cold water, such as salmon or mackerel. These contain a kind of fish oil that is good for your heart and actually lowers your cholesterol. Chicken and other poultry are good neutral foods; they have less fat although still some cholesterol. There is even less fat if you remove the skin. Monosaturated fats, such as olive oil, peanut oil, and rapeseed oil, are actually good for you. The official national nutritional guidelines call for a substitution of complex carbohydrates (such as whole wheat grains and cereals) for some of your fat intake and some of your protein intake.

What about other ways to lower your serum cholesterol and other blood lipids? There are some, and they are worth considering as you put together your own dietary plan. Fiber (as in celery, apples, beans, whole wheat grains, breads, and cereals) actually acts to lower cholesterol, as does Metamucil, by binding some cholesterol in the bowel. Adequate calcium intake, needed for strong bones, also lowers blood pressure and probably the blood lipids. Your exercise program lowers your total cholesterol and also increases the good HDL lipids in your blood. When you stop smoking, the HDL goes up. Good health habits all seem to fit together.

What about fish oil capsules? These contain the good fish oils such as those found in salmon and mackerel. Five capsules is about equivalent to one serving of salmon. They cost less than salmon. Thus there is nothing really wrong with using them, but in general we're not much for pills. These are big capsules, hard to swallow, and the process is a bit artificial. Besides, cats may start to follow you around.

What about taking one tablet of aspirin every other day to thin the blood? This should not replace dietary change and may not even be a good idea. Despite the publicity, studies on the subject should be considered preliminary. There has been no difference in deaths between subjects taking aspirin every other day and controls. There was a decrease in heart attacks, but this was compensated by increases in other categories of sudden death, including strokes. We believe that this regimen should be undertaken only with your doctor's advice. The same recommendation holds for the new cholesterol-lowering drugs as well as the old ones like niacin and cholestyramine. Try diet first, diet second, and diet third. Medication is fourth, if your doctor agrees.

SALT

Too much sodium in the system tends to retain fluid in the body, increasing the blood pressure and predisposing to problems such as swelling of the legs. The heart has to work harder with the increased amount of blood volume. Thus it is good to decrease salt intake. The average American takes in about 12 grams of sodium each day, one of the highest intakes in the world. Our convenience foods and our fast foods are usually loaded with salt. Salt is in ketchup, most sauces, and in hidden form in many foods. You need to read the labels to find it: Look for "sodium," not "salt." The recommended amount is 4 grams a day of salt for the typical person. You get plenty without adding anything. Under a doctor's advice, patients with problems of high blood pressure or heart failure or some other difficulties may need to reduce salt much more radically.

Do you have the typical American craving for junk foods? Don't despair—there are healthy snacks! Some of our favorites: popcorn, butterless, hot-air cooked, sprayed with butter-flavored PAM, and sprinkled with a little Parmesan cheese. Even better, try popcorn with olive oil instead of butter. Unsalted peanuts in the shell. French bread basted with olive oil and toasted with oregano or garlic.

FIBER

Adequate fiber intake is one of the latest popular health measures. It is much more than a fad. Fiber is the indigestible residue of food that passes through the entire bowel and is then eliminated in the stool. It is found in unrefined grains, cereals, vegetables (particularly celery), and some fruits. The beneficial aspects of high fiber intake come from its actions as it passes through the bowel. It attracts water and provides consistency to the stool so that it can pass easily. The resulting increased regularity of bowel action turns out to be very important. It decreases the chances of diverticulitis, an inflammation of the colon wall, which results from excessive pressure in the colon and weakening of the wall. It protects the bowel so that the development of precancerous polyps is greatly reduced, as is the risk of cancer of the colon. It also acts to decrease problems with constipation, hemorrhoids, tears in the rectal wall, and other minor problems as well as the big ones. It binds cholesterol and helps eliminate it from the body.

It needs to be emphasized that the natural fiber approach to regularity of the bowel is *greatly* to be preferred over use of laxatives and bowel stimulants, which have none of the above advantages. You need to get the fiber habit and avoid the laxative habit.

CALCIUM

Everybody needs enough calcium. This is particularly important for seniors and even more important for senior women. Our national trend toward better health habits has decreased intake of calcium-containing milk and cheese; hence, calcium intake for many people has dropped below what is desirable. Calcium supplements are often needed. Senior women should have at least 1,500 mg of calcium each day and men at least 1,000. A glass of milk (make it nonfat) contains about 250 mg of calcium. Add in the odds and ends of calcium in various foods, and a typical daily intake is usually around 500 mg. Hence most people need supplementation with calcium carbonate. The most popular forms are Tums and Oscal. Each tablet contains 500 mg. One or two tablets a day will usually do it. The reasons for maintaining calcium intake are discussed in a bit more detail in Chapter 15.

Remember the calcium "paradox," because it is important. Just taking calcium in your diet doesn't really do anything. The reason is that the calcium is not, for the most part, absorbed from the bowel. You need both to take enough calcium *and* to provide the body a stimulus to *absorb* the calcium from the bowel. For everybody, this stimulus should include weight-bearing exercise. For women, estrogen supplementation can be helpful, and this possible treatment should be discussed with your doctor.

SMOKING

Cigarette smoking kills 307,000 people in the United States each year, and most of these people are seniors. Lung cancer and emphysema are the best-known miserable outcomes. However, accelerated development of atherosclerosis is the most important problem resulting from smoking. This results in heart attacks and strokes, angina pectoris (heart pains), intermittent claudication (leg pains), and many other problems. Pipe and cigar smoking does not have the pulmonary (lung) consequences that cigarette smoking does, but does predispose to cancer of the lips, tongue, and esophagus. Nicotine in any form has the same bad effects on the small blood vessels and thus upon development of atherosclerosis.

It is never too late to quit. Only two years after stopping cigarette smoking, your risk of heart attack returns to average. It has actually decreased substantially the very next day! Most seniors have plenty of time to get major health benefits. After ten years your risk for lung cancer is back to nearly normal. After only two years, there is a decrease in lung cancer risk by perhaps one-third. The development of emphysema is arrested for many people when they stop smoking, although this does not reverse.

Seniors often feel that it is too late for changes in lifestyle to have beneficial effects on their health. Not so—chances of stroke and heart attack begin to go down immediately. Moreover, you will notice at once that your environment has become more friendly when you are not a smoker. Many of the daily hassles that impair the quality of your life go away when you stop offending others by this habit.

Here are some tips for quitting: Decide firmly that you really want to do it. You need to believe that you can do it. Set a date on which you will stop smoking. Announce this date to your friends. When the day comes, stop. You can expect that the physical addiction to nicotine may make you nervous and irritable for a period of about 48 hours. After that, there is no further *physical* addiction. There is, of course, the psychological craving, which sometimes lasts a very long period of time. Often, however, it is quite short. Reward yourself every week or so with something nice that you have bought with what would have been cigarette money. Combine your stop-smoking program with an increase in your exercise program. The two changes fit together naturally. Exercise will take your mind off the smoking change, and it will decrease the tendency to gain weight in the early weeks after stopping smoking; this is the only negative consequence of stopping. The immediate rewards include better-tasting food, truer friends, less cough, better stamina, more money, fewer holes in your clothes, and membership in a larger world.

Many health educators are skeptical about cutting down slowly and stress that you need to stop completely. We don't think this is always true for seniors. For some people rationing is a good way to get their smoking down to a much lower level and then at that point it may be easier to stop entirely. For example, the simple decision not to smoke in public can help both your health and decrease your daily hassles. To cut down, only keep in the cigarette pack those cigarettes that you are going to allow yourself that day. Smoke the cigarettes only halfway down before extinguishing them.

There are now many good stop-smoking courses being offered through the Cancer Society, the Lung Association, or your local hospital. Most people actually don't need these, but if you do, they can help you be successful. Try by yourself first. Then, if you still need help, there is a lot of it around.

Nicotine chewing gum can help some people quit, and your doctor can give you a prescription and advice. Don't plan on this as a long-term solution, since the nicotine in the gum is just as bad for your arteries as is the nicotine in cigarettes.

An example of your ability to make your own choices is afforded by the challenge to stop smoking. If you are trapped by your addictions, even the lesser ones, you can't make your own choices. Victory over smoking behaviors improves your mental health, in part because this is a difficult victory. It can open the door to success in other areas.

Alcohol

Excessive alcohol intake is not often a major problem for seniors. Most seniors who drink are moderate in their habit. Moderate drinkers actually appear to have slightly better health overall than those who don't drink any alcohol at all. The heavy drinkers, with cirrhosis and other major medical problems, usually haven't survived to their senior years.

Of course, excessive alcohol intake is a problem for some people in every age group. With seniors the most frequent problem is that excessive drinking leads to depression, and this can have negative effects on your entire life. Seniors should look for the same danger signs as do younger individuals. These include morning drinking, citations for driving while intoxicated, automobile accidents after any alcohol intake at all, drinking to make problems go away, drinking behavior that worries your spouse or your friends, medical problems of ulcer or gastritis. If any of these danger signs have occurred in your recent life, you should cut down. If more than one of them has occurred, you should contact your nearest Alcoholic Anonymous chapter or get some other form of professional help.

Even if your drinking is moderate, occasional, and purely social, remember still that alcohol is a drug. As with other drugs, you cannot tolerate as large a dose as you could when you were younger. You may find that alcohol aggravates your sleeping patterns or that you cannot tolerate certain kinds of alcohol such as red wine or straight hard liquor. White wine and light beers are among the easiest forms of alcohol to tolerate as you grow older.

Obesity

Excessive body weight compounds many health problems. It stresses the heart, the muscles, and the bones. It increases the likelihood of hernias, hemorrhoids, gallbladder disease, varicose veins, and many other things. Excess weight makes breathing more difficult. Additional weight slows you down, makes you less effective in personal encounters, and lowers your self-image. Fat people are hospitalized more frequently than people with normal weight; they have more gallbladder problems, more surgical complications, more cases of breast cancer, more high blood pressure, more heart attacks, and more strokes.

Weight control is a difficult task. Fortunately, it becomes a little easier for seniors than for others. Maximum body weights are generally obtained between 45 and 64 years of age; after this most individuals do lose some weight. Excess weight is very seldom due to thyroid disease or other specific illness that causes a problem of overweight. For most of us the problem and the solution are personal, not medical. As with the other habits that change health, management of this problem begins with its recognition as a problem. Weight control requires continued attention. For those of us with a potential problem, the vigilance must be lifelong.

Increasingly, exercise is being seen as an important key to weight control. Part of every weight control program should be an exercise program. Obesity is not just the result of overeating. Obese people, when studied carefully, are found to move around less and therefore to burn too few calories. If you burn too few calories and take in just an average amount, you will gain weight. There is nothing very mysterious about calories. Thirty-five hundred calories equals about a pound of body weight. If you take in 3,500 calories less than you burn, you lose a pound. If you take in 3,500 more than you burn, you gain a pound. If you want your horse to lose weight, you just give him less hay or exercise him more.

There are two important phases to weight control: the *weight reduction* phase and the *weight maintenance* phase. The weight reduction phase is the easiest. Here, the method you use to lose weight doesn't matter too much, although you should check with your doctor if you plan to lose a large amount of weight quickly to make sure that the diet you intend is a sound one. During the weight loss stage, many of your calories are provided by your own body fat and protein as they are being broken down, so you need little or no fat and much less protein in your diet during this period. Complex carbohydrates are important to most sound diets. Diets usually have a gimmick of some kind that encourages you and helps you remember the diet.

Most people have some success in losing weight. If you set a target, tell people what you are trying to do, and stick with it for a while, you can probably lose weight. Remember that it has to go slowly, however, since even a total fast will cause true weight loss of less than a pound a day. Rapid changes in weight are generally due to loss of fluid. Because low-calorie diets tend to be lower in salt, the first few days of a diet give you a false sense of accomplishment as you lose some of the fluid that the salt was retaining in your body. Then, when the rate of weight loss slows down, you may think that the diet has failed. You have to be patient with the weight loss phase. A pound a week is a reasonable goal. This requires elimination of the equivalent of one day's food each week.

The second phase is *maintenance* of weight at the desirable weight you have now achieved. This is more difficult, and it requires constant attention. Weigh yourself regularly and record the weight on a chart. Draw a red line at three pounds over your desired weight and maintain the weight below the line, using whatever method works best for you. Accept no excuses for increasing weight; it is easier and healthier to make frequent small adjustments in what you eat than to try and counteract binges of overeating with dieting. Keep yourself off the dietary roller coaster.

Other Health Habits

An old joke maintains that everything that is pleasurable is either illegal, immoral, or fattening. This is exactly the wrong idea. Health is pleasurable; ill health is miserable. Good health habits are their own immediate reward. If changes toward healthier behaviors are making you feel less well, you are doing something wrong. Exercise makes you feel better. Good diets make you feel better. Nicotine avoidance makes you feel better. Having a good body weight makes your life activities easier and more pleasurable.

Much that is written about healthy behaviors makes the whole process seem mysterious and complicated. The tabloids in supermarket magazines are always reporting some new threat to your health. Here we have tried to emphasize only the important and the proven. Only five areas require your attention: *exercise, diet, smoking cessation, alcohol moderation,* and *weight control.*

There is a long list of other possible threats to health, but they have two problems: First, they often are not adequately proven. Second, even if they do prove to be true, they aren't very important compared with the big five discussed above. Fix these five first. Common sense can help you keep your priorities right. We do suggest moderation in barbecued foods because of possible carcinogenesis, but only if you are having such meals more than 30 times a year. And many people will find their life more pleasant if they control their caffeine intake, particularly in the evening. Even these problems are not very scientifically well established, and changes here are of much less importance than changes in the five major areas.

CHAPTER 8

The Doctor

The times have changed. We grew up with "doctor knows best," the view that the doctor represents knowledge and authority and everyone else follows "doctor's orders." Now it is recognized that the best health results from a working partnership between doctor and patient. The doctor brings information and experience, you bring your own values and your own goals. The therapeutic plan is negotiated between the two partners. After hearing the doctor's perspective on your problems and their potential solutions, you make the choice. It is very important at this time of your life that you have the right doctor.

Choosing the Right Doctor

You should have one personal physician in whom you have trust and confidence. This physician should be your advocate and your guide through the complicated medical care system. A consultant may be required from time to time, and his or her recommendations should be interpreted and coordinated by your personal doctor. Good medical care usually does not result from an arrangement whereby you have a different doctor for every organ of your body. Someone has to have the whole picture, to know everything that is going on. Having too many doctors working in an uncoordinated manner often results in too many medications, too many medical procedures, too many side effects, and sometimes in contradictory approaches to treatment. Your personal doctor doesn't need to be an expert in everything; he or she should readily seek advice from others when needed. He or she can help guide you to other appropriate health professionals. Someone needs to take responsibility for putting all the information together and making sure that nothing has been left out.

What kind of a physician should your personal physician be? He or she might appropriately be a family practitioner (specialist in family medicine), an internist (specialist in internal medicine), or a geriatrician (specialist in the medical care of older people). The family practitioner and the general internist are trained in dealing with the "whole patient" and in appropriate use of other consultants as required. Geriatrics is a relatively new specialty with practice limited to the senior population, and its practitioners take pride in recognizing the needs of the whole patient as well. Most internal medicine problems now occur after the age of 65, so the general internist has become, in large part, a geriatrician.

Often, your primary doctor should be a specialist! Does this sound contradictory? Not if you have a particular medical problem. If you anticipate that over one-half of your medical problems over the next several years are going to be in a particular specialty area, you may want to find a specialist in that area who will also take responsibility for coordinating other care you might need. If most of your problems are gynecological, you might want a gynecologist to be your personal physician. If you have rheumatoid arthritis, you may wish a rheumatologist to be your primary physician. If you have had two heart attacks and are suffering from angina pectoris, a cardiologist might be your best choice. If you already have a defined major problem, it makes good sense to receive guidance on that problem from people who know the most about it. You need expert help.

In this situation it becomes inefficient to have a general physician who always has to refer you to the specialist. As noted above, it is not a good idea to have two or more primary physicians at the same time.

Table 8–1 notes some of the attributes that you will want in a primary care physician. Note that these attributes center around *communication* and *anticipation*. A good doctor will listen carefully to you and will explain his or her suggested course of action clearly. Prevention of future problems will be a substantial part of the conversation. Problems will be anticipated and plans made before the problems become severe. This includes anticipation of possible side effects from medication, as well as considering specific diseases that may be avoided by particular actions. A good doctor is available to you (or has provided alternatives) in the office, over the phone, and at home.

The physician needs your trust and confidence. If you can't communicate with a particular doctor, try another. Often the failed communication really isn't anyone's fault; two people may just happen to be operating on different frequencies. You want to keep the same doctor for a long period of time. So if a relationship with a particular physician is not working out, change, but change early. When you find the right doctor, stay with that physician unless there is a substantial change in your medical needs that requires a doctor with different skills.

TABLE 8.1. *Attributes of Your Primary Physician*

Takes time to talk
Takes time to listen
Plans ahead to prevent problems
Prescribes medication carefully and reluctantly
Reviews total program regularly
Is available by phone
Has your trust and confidence
Makes house calls

Communication is the human side of medicine, and it is more important than ever. In an age of chronic illness in which preventive factors are so important and medication represents a two-edged sword, you need a doctor you can talk with and whom you can understand.

There is a technical side of medicine too, and for many individuals this will represent the most important part of modern medicine. Perhaps you need an operation on your blood vessels or your brain. Perhaps you need surgery inside your middle ear. Perhaps you need replacement of your right hip, you require kidney dialysis, or you need an organ transplant. In these situations your criteria for excellence in your consulting physician are a little different. You are still interested in anticipation and communication, but you also want to pay a great deal of attention to the *technical skill* of the individual.

You would like to know if this particular surgeon, for example, gets better or worse results than average. This is often a little hard to judge, but there are two key tests that you can apply. First, does the specialist have the complete confidence and approval of your primary physician? Talk with your primary physician about possible alternatives, and ask about the advantages and disadvantages of each. Second, ask how frequently the specialist performs the particular procedure. Technical results are generally better at institutions and with physicians who perform the procedure frequently. As a general rule, results are substantially better where the procedure is done 50 times or more each year, and less good where the procedure is only done occasionally.

The above considerations do not apply only to surgical specialists. Increasingly the line between surgery and medicine has become blurred. There are now "invasive cardiologists" who perform marvelous but sometimes hazardous tasks through long tubes manipulated through your blood vessels under x-ray control. The gastrointestinal "endoscopist" can now use long, flexible lighted tubes to look at (and sometimes treat) a surprising amount of your insides from the outside. An arthroscopist can perform surgery inside the joint with only a small cut in the skin required to admit a lighted tube with which to see the inside of the joint. Arteriographers, often radiologists, use dye injected through long catheters to visualize your blood vessels on x-ray. New x-ray techniques include computed tomography and nuclear magnetic resonance imagery. These techniques require skill both for performing the procedure and for interpretation of the results. Again, apply your two tests. Does the specialist who will do the procedure have the full agreement and confidence of your primary physician? Does the specialist perform the procedure frequently?

Negotiating a Plan

Working out your plan for aging well will include your doctor's help. The old rituals of medicine with the authoritative physician and the passive patient are undergoing reevaluation. In the old relationship, the doctor would ask a series of questions, and you answered. The doctor then carefully examined all parts of your body. Then the doctor ordered tests. Then you were given a prescription and you left. These traditional parts of the physician–patient encounter are still important, but they are no longer enough, by themselves, and they should not monopolize all the available time during your encounter.

You need to talk, too. You need to ask what to anticipate and how to prevent problems. You need to discuss your goals and values. The doctor needs to know how you feel about treatment of your symptoms versus the side effects that might come from treatment.

You don't want to limit a valuable physician encounter only to your current problems. You may have a lot of questions. The physician visit is a good place to begin thinking, together with a knowledgable professional, about solutions. (A list of possible discussion areas is shown in Table 8–2.) You also want

TABLE 8.2. *Some Subjects to Discuss*

Exercise
Diet
Calcium
Estrogen for women
Mammography for women
Sexual problems
Weight control
Smoking
Drug or alcohol habituation
Medication program

TABLE 8.3. *A Question List*

What is my problem?
What is wrong with me?
Is it a common problem?
What does the diagnosis mean?
Can you tell me what the words (any words you don't understand) mean?
Could the problem be anything else?
How likely is that?
What do I need to do now?
What should I do at home?
Is there anything I shouldn't do?
When should I check back with you?

If tests are ordered:
What will be learned by these tests?
Should I expect any discomfort from them?
Do I need to make special arrangements (such as fasting before the test or planning transportation home)?

If medication is prescribed:
Is there any alternative to taking this medication?
How does the medication help?
Does it have any side effects I should know about?
Is it available in a generic form?
Are there interactions with other drugs or with foods?

What can I expect in the next few weeks and also over the long term?

What are the risks of this procedure?
How frequently does this procedure relieve my problem?
Must the procedure be done right away?
If it has to be done right away, why?
How frequently do you do this procedure?
I would feel more comfortable with another opinion. Could you recommend someone for me to check with?
Can this procedure be done safely as an outpatient?

to make the doctor's time count. You may only have a few minutes. You want the doctor to be efficient during his or her time with you so that you can get the most out of it.

To use time effectively, make a list of your questions before the doctor visit and take it with you. Write out your questions on a piece of paper. Date the list. Leave space to jot down answers while you are talking with the doctor. If someone is accompanying you on the visit, perhaps he or she can write down the answers for you. Ask the doctor each question. Go over the list and the answers again after you get home. Save the list as part of your own records.

Table 8–3 give you some suggestions for questions that you may want to include on your list. Run through this list and see which questions you may want to include as you make up your list for a particular visit. There are many other questions that you may want to include as well, but the table can help you get started.

The next table (Table 8–4) shows what the list might look like for a visit to Dr. Johanson because of a problem with dizziness when standing up. Your list on the left will probably be handwritten and the answers on the right jotted down, but this example will give you a general idea of the process.

The Checkup

The value of "checkups" has often been overstated in recent years. Indiscriminate "fishing" for minor abnormalities is not often helpful. Early *detection* programs should be directed at potential problems that have three characteristics. First, the potential problem should be an *important* one, not just some minor laboratory abnormality you don't even need to know about. Second, the problem should be *asymptomatic* (not causing symptoms). If it is already causing symptoms, you should have been including the symptoms on your list, and the investigation should

TABLE 8.4. *Problem List for Dr. Johanson, March 17, 1989*

Questions	*Answers*
1. Dizziness when standing?	**Low blood pressure. Decrease Aldomet to two a day. Will check blood counts.**
2. Wonder about aspirin or fish oil capsules for heart attacks?	**Not yet. Diet first. Will check cholesterol.**
3. Leg cramps at night.	**Warm baths and massage.**
4. Gray splotches on skin.	**Just age spots. OK.**
5. Move to Arizona for joint pains.	**Probably not. Try a vacation to a hot, dry area first, see if feel better.**
6. Cost of blood pressure pills.	**Reducing dose anyway because of dizziness. Try AARP pharmacy services.**

proceed from that point. Third, the potential condition must be *treatable*. That is, there must be an effective treatment available if an important abnormality is found. Not very many "checkup" procedures pass all three of these tests.

On the other hand, *checkups are more important for seniors than for younger individuals*. Checkups can help you set your health agenda. You are at higher risk for most diseases, so the yield of the search is greater. Checkups can reveal some important things that you didn't know about, and sometimes identification of these things can be lifesaving.

An important example is high blood pressure. High blood pressure can exist for a long time and cause accelerated damage to your blood vessels before you have any symptoms at all. If you know about your high blood pressure, you can develop a program to eliminate most of the later complications. Similarly, early detection of a number of cancers can be lifesaving. Breast cancer, colon and rectal cancer, cancer of the uterine cervix, and cancer of the body of the uterus can often be detected before you have any symptoms. Important clues can come from blood tests that assess the function of your kidneys or from the finding of blood in your stool or abnormalities in your urine on urinalysis. Your doctor can assist you by recommending specific tests that may be of help and suggesting the frequency with which such tests should be performed.

The National Blue Cross and Blue Shield Association has recently reviewed reports from various committees that have investigated the usefulness of screening procedures and the frequency with which they should be performed. We like their recommendations (shown in Table 8–5), since they represent a current consensus, emphasize the important test procedures, and don't overdo the recommendations for routine screening.

TABLE 8.5. *Your Schedule for Checkups (Modified Recommendations for Over Age 65)*

For Cervical Cancer in Women

Pap smear every two years

For Colorectal Cancer

Fecal occult blood tests every year

Sigmoidoscopy every three to five years, yearly if abnormal

Air-contrast barium enema every three to five years if there has been colon cancer in a parent or sibling

For Breast Cancer in Women

Monthly breast self-examination

Physical examination and mammography yearly

For Lung Cancer

Screening with chest x-rays or sputum cytology is not recommended

For Asymptomatic Coronary Artery Disease

Exercise stress testing is not recommended

Resting electrocardiogram is not recommended

For Cardiac Risk Factors

Serum Cholesterol every five years

Blood pressure check yearly

For Diabetes

Screening for diabetes is not recommended

For Osteoporosis

Screening for osteoporosis is not recommended

Not all physicians will agree with every recommendation, but these provide a good basic overview.

Many people feel that there can't be any danger with using screening tests more frequently than this, but they neglect to consider the problems that occur with overscreening. With most of these screening tests, "false-positive" results are much more common than "true-positive" results. In other words, many of the things that are picked up by the tests aren't really there. But, when a possible abnormality is found, it is usually necessary to follow up on it. This may involve a series of other tests, and these tests are not only expensive, but they often carry some degree of risk. They can lead to psychological discomfort, unnecessary hospitalization or even unnecessary surgery. Or there can be a serious side effect from the diagnostic test itself.

Thus you can run into problems either way. If you don't find an asymptomatic condition early enough, you might develop a progressive condition and have a bad medical result. On the other hand, if testing suggests the presence of a problem that you really don't have, you can get into problems that way. Different people may well have different priorities, some being more worried by the possibility of disease and others by the possibility of expensive and unnecessary procedures. If you have been following the general recommendations of this chapter, you have a primary physician in whom you have trust and confidence and with whom you can discuss such issues comfortably. If you have questions about screening and checkups, put them on the list.

CHAPTER 9

Medications

A good part of aging well is moderation and caution in the use of medications. *Seniors eliminate drugs from their body slowly and usually need only relatively low doses.* We have all grown up with medicines and they are part of us. They can be lifesaving. They can modify serious diseases. They can help us endure bothersome symptoms. But there is a dark side to the miracles of modern medicine. Some 10 to 20 percent of hospitalizations for seniors are the result of drug side effects. These can largely be prevented. Each year 2,000,000,000 prescriptions are written in the United States. This is eight prescriptions per year for every man, women, and child. Seniors average over 12 prescriptions per year per person. It is not surprising that problems sometimes occur with such widespread use. You need to balance the good that drugs do against their potential harm.

Your Defense Mechanisms

The body is designed to defend itself against outside threats (such as bacteria) and to heal itself after injury. It does so by using its own "defense mechanisms," some of which are listed in Table 9–1. However, because of our emphasis upon medical cure and alleviation of symptoms, we sometimes mistake these defense mechanisms for diseases in their own right. Many medications actually act to block defense mechanisms. This may result in the body being unable to cope as effectively with another problem.

For example, when we *cough*, infectious particles are cleared from our lungs so that we can breathe better. This is the "good" part of a cough. Usually we don't want to suppress a cough that is eliminating bad materials from the body, since this can result in the infection staying in the lungs. The common *sneeze* clears particles that can cause allergic reactions from the respiratory system. In the mucus of a *runny nose* are special antibodies that attach to attacking virus particles and carry them outside the body so that the viral infection is not as serious. *Diarrhea* helps to remove toxins and bacteria from the bowels so that they can't cause as much illness. If we block the diarrhea, the body might absorb these toxins. *Fever* helps speed up the body's actions in order to fight infection by increasing blood flow and metabolic rates. *Pain* is a great aid to us over the long run, even though it hurts. It helps protect injured body parts by encouraging us not to move them much until they heal, and it signals us to rapidly remove our hand from a hot object. *Inflammation* is a natural part of the healing process of the body. This process

TABLE 9.1. *Your Defense Mechanisms*

Symptom	*Positive Action*
Cough	**Clears infection from the lungs**
Sneeze	**Clears allergy particles**
Runny nose	**Takes virus outside body**
Diarrhea	**Removes toxins and bacteria from the bowels**
Fever	**Speeds up the body to fight infection**
Pain	**Protects injured body parts**
Inflammation	**Necessary to heal injury or damage**

clears away the damaged materials and brings new materials to the injured site to facilitate repair. Defense mechanisms are part of the "wisdom of the body."

This is not to say that we should *never* use medication for defense mechanism symptoms. It does mean that you should think very carefully when you hear about medications that promise "instant relief." Usually this approach treats only the symptoms, not the disease. Doctors have been gradually modifying their approach toward treatment of common symptoms, relying more on time and the natural healing powers of the body and less on symptomatic medications. With time, most things get better. Thus, diarrhea is now treated more frequently with antibiotics and increased fluid intake than by drugs (such as Lomotil and Kaopectate) that slow down the bowel activity. Fever is not generally suppressed unless it is quite high. Pain medications now are used with caution unless the injured part is simultaneously immobilized by casting or splinting. Coughs are treated by use of expectorants that increase the mucus and fluid production rather than by drugs such as codeine that suppress the cough reflex. Try to be cautious in your own self-medication, and if there are questions, take them up with your doctor, at least by telephone. We advise frequently reviewing your entire medication program with your doctor so as to keep the list of drugs taken as small as possible and we suggest that you personally use over-the-counter medications as sparingly as possible.

The Declining Dose Requirement—A Central Principle

As we age, our bodies eliminate medications from our bodies at a slower rate. In medical terms, the drug is "metabolized" more slowly with age. Drugs are usually eliminated by the liver and kidney, and these organs work more slowly when you are older. Thus a small dose of medication goes a long way. In essence, we can get the same good effect for a lower dosage when we are older, while on the other hand, the "regular" dose of a drug can become an overdose. The first rule of medication use in older individuals is to keep the dose appropriately low.

In older patients, a small dose of codeine may cause severe fatigue and sleepiness. A little digitalis may cause profound nausea and vomiting; a diuretic to remove fluid from the ankles may cause dizziness and kidney problems. Or, entirely new side effects can appear in the elderly. A sleeping pill can keep the patient awake. A tranquilizer may excite the patient or cause severe depression. Your central rule: Work with your doctor to keep doses as appropriately low as possible, and quickly consider that any new problem that arises *might* be a problem resulting from a medication.

Table 9–2 lists some common side effects and some of the drugs that can cause them. This is a very partial list. In the "package insert" list of drug side effects that physicians use, most medications are recognized to cause 20 or more different side effects on occasion. This doesn't mean that everybody

TABLE 9.2. *Some Common Side Effects*

Symptom	*Responsible Drug*
Drowsiness	**Antihistamines, codeine, tranquilizers, sedatives**
Nausea	**Almost anything on occasion**
Ulcers	**Aspirin, Advil, Nuprin, other antiinflammatory drugs**
Dizziness	**High blood pressure drugs, many others**
Bleeding	**Aspirin, Coumadin, heparin**
Bruising	**Aspirin, prednisone**
Rash	**Antibiotics, almost anything on occasion**
Memory loss/confusion	**Tranquilizers, codeine, sedatives, antihistamines**
Fluid retention	**Antiinflammatory drugs, prednisone, many others**
Diarrhea	**Some antacids, almost anything on occasion**

gets these side effects; indeed, some of them are very unusual. Most of the time when a side effect is encountered, it will go away quite rapidly when the drug is discontinued. So, you need to be alert to this possible problem—it often has a very easy solution.

Multiple Problems and Multiple Medications

Most of the major diseases of our time are more common in the older patient—diabetes, atherosclerosis, osteoarthritis, cancer. The older patient commonly will have several problems at once, thus creating special difficulties. If you already have one significant medical problem, a second one is more serious than if it occurred when you were in good health. This is another reason why you want to prevent as many problems as possible *before* they occur.

One problem can easily complicate another. High blood pressure can increase kidney failure, which can increase blood pressure. A problem of breathlessness caused by the heart can complicate breathlessness caused by lung disease. Arthritis can increase inactivity, which can lead to blood clots in the legs. Your approach to these problems sometimes must be a compromise after all aspects of the situation are considered. You need a doctor to help you in such decisions much more often than in the uncomplicated isolated illnesses of relative youth.

The older patient is frequently taking a number of different medications, often on elaborate schedules. In medical slang, using too many medications is termed "polypharmacy." A patient may be taking a diuretic (water pill) for swelling of the legs, a medication to help eliminate the uric acid caused by the water pill, a tranquilizer for anxiety, a sedative to sleep, an antacid to settle the stomach, a hormone to replace lost glandular functions, a pain medication for arthritis, an antiinflammatory agent for muscle aches, a laxative to help elimination, miscellaneous vitamins and minerals, iron for the blood, and additional medications whenever a new problem comes up. This is an especially common scenario in older patients, and usually the use of the many drugs has built up over a long time. Often, the physician prescribing a new agent is not even aware of the long list of drugs already being taken.

The side effects of these many medications add up and may cause illness. Even more importantly, the drugs may intefere with each other. Sedatives can dangerously slow the metabolism of Coumadin, a blood-thinning drug. The action of the uric acid drug may be blocked by aspirin. Antacids can decrease the effectiveness of antibiotics. Antiinflammatory drugs can cause retention of fluid, which then requires a water pill or diuretic. The interactions between different drugs when multiple medications are taken become so complicated that no physician or scientist fully understands them.

Use as few drugs as possible. Obviously, no harmful drug interactions can occur if only a single drug is taken. This is not possible for all patients at all times, but if your drug intake is kept minimal, your doctor can usually help you find combinations of medications that are known to work well together.

Cutting Back

Follow these three general principles:

1. *Avoid tranquilizers* (nerve pills), *sedatives* (sleeping pills), *and analgesics* (pain pills) *whenever possible.* These drugs have many bad effects and often do not solve the problem.

2. Use lifestyle change instead of medication *whenever possible.* Avoiding salt in your diet is better than taking a "water pill." Exercise programs can reduce the need for blood pressure medications, and weight reduction will usually work better than pills for diabetes. There are many other examples listed throughout this book.

3. *Get rid of the "optional" medications.* Crucial drugs make up less than 10 percent of all prescriptions in the United States. Over-the-counter drugs are completely at your option. Almost by definition these drugs are not crucial. If you started them without the advice of your physician, you can stop them without the advice of your physician.

In addition to tranquilizers, sedatives, and minor pain medications, drugs that are often optional include allopurinol (Zyloprim) given for serum uric acid elevation without gout, diuretics (water pills) given for "fluid retention" in the absence of an actual disease, hormonal supplements that are not related to a disease, and pills (oral hypoglycemics) given for adult-onset diabetes. There are many other optional drugs. This is not to say that these drugs are not beneficial on occasion, but more often they are not necessary. The decision to use them must be made with caution, and that decision must be reviewed periodically.

Vitamins and Minerals

It has been said that Americans have the "most expensive urine in the world" because they so frequently take unneeded vitamins and minerals, which are then rapidly excreted by the body in the urine, without gain. Unless you have an unusual medical condition or eat a very unbalanced diet, you do not need vitamin supplements. If you have pernicious anemia, you may need vitamin B_{12} shots; vitamin D is sometimes prescribed for severe osteoporosis; iron and other minerals may be needed on occasion; and folic acid is needed once in a while for another kind of anemia. Other than this kind of unusual problem, vitamins are optional.

I don't think that routine vitamin use makes much sense, and claims for extra energy or fewer colds are not scientifically founded. On the other hand, I don't think that vitamin supplements or even "megavitamin" programs do much harm, as a rule. Only vitamins A and D are likely to be toxic in large doses. Iron can cause severe constipation. There is more emotionalism about vitamins than about almost any subject, and if someone tells me that they are benefiting from a particular vitamin program, I try not to discourage him or her. Generally, the potential harm of unneeded vitamin intake involves only the unnecessary cost of the vitamins and the possibility that needed medical care may not be undertaken because of the assumption that the vitamins are enough.

You do have to be aware of hoaxes that use vitamins as gimmicks. In these promotions the "secret tonic" may be vitamins, minerals, or Gerovital, but the sales pitch is the same. You need this special secret tonic. Incidentally, the "snake oil" seller gets your money.

A typical example is Laetrile, a purported cancer treatment. Laetrile is not actually a vitamin but has been promoted as one. Usually, it has been offered as part of an exploitation scheme. While medical authorities have raised alarms over the small amount of cyanide contained in Laetrile, its real harm comes from the theft of dignity. It is difficult enough to deal with a cancer without spending the last few days of your life realizing that you were deluded by a swindle. Scientific evidence that this agent is not effective in treatment of any form of cancer is now conclusive.

The megavitamin craze appears to have passed its peak and to be subsiding. This has been a clever and novel way to sell large quantities of vitamins but has never had any real scientific support. Vitamin C, by the carload, has been the most imaginatively promoted. As evidence mounted that it did not help the common cold, it was advocated for cancer treatment.

As evidence grew that it didn't work there, it was touted as an arthritis cure. We have studied its effects in arthritis and can't find any.

Common sense is your best guide to vitamin use. A good, balanced diet is your best protection against vitamin deficiency.

A Word on Water

There *is* a master medicine. It is calorie-free, pure, contains no fat or cholesterol, and is best for you without any additives. It helps your kidneys flush out the bad humors. If you have a fever or the flu or if the weather is very hot, it can be lifesaving. The medicine is water. Cool, clear water. Drink a glass or more each day. With flu or hot weather take a goodly amount, in small amounts every few minutes. You should drink enough water so that at least once each day your urine is nearly colorless, and you should be voiding urine at least three times a day.

The Bottom Line

The bottom line is common sense. You need to respect drugs for the miracles that they can do. You have to be vigilant to the harm that may occur. You should make a list of all the medications you are currently using and take it with you on each doctor visit. Your program should be reviewed and any unnecessary drugs discontinued. With over-the-counter drugs, your own moderation is the important factor.

When any new problem arises, suspect first that it might be the result of a drug you are taking. This is the easiest of all medical problems to treat. You stop the drug, and generally the problem goes away.

With prescription drugs, don't stop them without talking with your physician, at least by phone, because you may not understand the full importance of that particular medication. Seek out a physician who views medication skeptically and with respect.

We do want to get all the substantial benefits from modern medications. This inevitably means that we will have some side effects. Often, we cannot tell in advance which patients are most likely to have the side reactions. But, if doses are kept appropriately low with regard to the age of the patient, and only necessary medications are employed, the risk is very much less.

Probably the 10 to 20 percent of senior hospitalizations currently related to drug side effects could be cut to perhaps 2 to 4 percent. Cautious and skeptical use of medications is a very important part of your personal program to age well.

CHAPTER 10

The Healthy Head

One of the great fears of growing older is the possibility of becoming senile and losing your mind. For the most part, this is another myth of aging, but every time we can't remember the right word or have trouble recalling something that we think we should know, we tend to worry. We think that perhaps this is a sign that our minds are getting old. In fact, senility is quite unusual, affecting only some 5 to 10 percent of individuals over the age of 85. The great majority of older individuals do *not* have fundamental organic problems with their minds.

Of course, there are some real difficulties. The speed at which nerve impulses are transmitted declines slowly with age, so thinking and remembering processes do tend to be a bit slower. And the accumulated store of memories is so much larger that it can take the brain longer to find a particular item. Moreover, there are small breaks scattered through the nerve connections in our brains, and these increase as we get older. This means that the nerve impulses need to take detours or establish new routes, and this also slows things down. But these are not really fundamental problems.

To a large extent, problems with memory and thinking are just the same as problems with our physical body. If we don't use a faculty, we will lose it. The myths of aging tend to make us expect intellectual decline. Actually, if we use our minds frequently and in novel ways, many of the attributes of intelligence, such as wisdom, actually can improve with age. Remember the analogy with your physical body, and think about "jogging" the memory, "exercising" the mind. The principles are the same as those of physical exercise, but the techniques are different. You need to understand a little bit about how the brain works and how you can work to improve its operation. Like any exercise, exercises for your intelligence can be a little uncomfortable, particularly at first. Like physical exercise, you need daily regular practice. You also need to select those areas that are most important to you to work on the hardest.

Jogging the Memory

To work on memory problems, you need to know about *short-term memory, long-term memory,* and about the concept of an *index.* When we are first presented with a new item, it goes into our short-term memory. The item can be presented through any of our senses. We can hear it, we can read about it, we can see it, we can feel it, or we can even smell it. Our *short-term memory,* however, is very small. It can hold only seven or eight chunks of data at a time and it only holds these for a few moments. Thus, we can usually remember a seven-digit number, like a telephone number, but if the number of chunks gets larger, we cannot hold it in short-term memory.

Our *long-term memory* includes the complicated storage of all the items of our experience. When we remember something, we remember it from the long-term memory storage place. To do this, we need an *index* that tells the brain where the item is stored so that it knows where to look to find it. Actually, we cross-index items many different ways. If we want to remember something about a canary, we may have it indexed under "birds." We probably also have it indexed under "yellow things." We might also have an item indexed with things that rhyme with it.

Table 10–1 indicates this sequence of memory and summarizes methods you can use for improvement at each step.

The memory problems that come with age are usually the result of a problem in one of three parts of this process. First, we may not concentrate on an item enough to even put it in our short-term memory. Thus you might be introduced to someone but not catch the name. Second, we may just let it fade out of short-term memory without ever storing it in our long-term memories. "I just met the man over there, but I can't remember his name." Third, we might have stored the item, but we have lost part of the index and have trouble finding it again. The index is reestablished and strengthened every time you use a particular memory path in your brain, but if you haven't used it for a while, there may be a break in the path. This results in the common phenomenon, "I can't remember it now, but wait a minute, it will come to me." This means that your direct index isn't working, and the brain has to do a lot of searching to find that particular item. Sometimes you won't find it until the next day until you will suddenly "remember" what you couldn't before.

TABLE 10.1. *Memory*

Process	*Treatment*
Short-term memory	**Concentration**
	Repetition
Long-term memory	**Association**
	Cue creation
Index	**Practice**
	Use
	Reuse
Retrieval	**Use**
	Reuse

To be sure that a new item is presented to your short-term memory, you need to be alert. You are most alert if you are free from medications that may impair your concentration, if your surroundings are quiet without distraction, and if your hearing, vision, and other senses are working correctly. Many "memory" problems are dramatically improved just by getting a hearing aid, by getting the right pair of glasses, or by having cataract surgery.

To move an item from short-term memory to long-term memory, the primary technique is repetition. "Use it five times and it's yours." Repetition should be immediate, and also it should be further repeated over the first 24 hours for best results. At the same time, associating the new item with other items will help your recall. You will also help to build your indexing structures by association.

The index to long-term memory has to do with the creation of memory cues. These require associations of a new item with older items and organization of a logical memory path to find the item within your brain.

The index is under continual attack from little physical breaks, and constantly needs to be reestablished. It may take some time to find a particular memory that we have not visited in a long time. The next day we can find that same memory more quickly. Recent practice and use and reuse of our memory pathways keep them well established and intact. Thus if we only use a few of our memory pathways, the others fall into disrepair and our overall intelligence becomes unnecessarily limited.

The introduction sequence described in the box summarizes the techniques for placing a new item in long-term memory. A new person is introduced. The listener pays careful attention to the name, and further concentrates by asking for the spelling. She associates the name with the person by referring to a typewriter company of the same name, his dwelling, his occupation, by careful attention to his physical features, by noting his height, and by concentrating on the content of his conversation.

Remembering a Name

"This is Mr. John Underwood"

"I'm very pleased to meet you, Mr. Underward. Tell me, how do you spell your last name?"

"U-N-D-E-R-W-O-O-D."

"That's an interesting name. I used to have an Underwood typewriter. Where do you live, Mr. Underwood? What kind of work do you do?"

(Five minutes later)

"Joan, I want you to meet Mr. John Underwood. He lives over on Linden Street, and used to work as an accountant." (Looks again closely at Mr. Underwood.)

(30 minutes later)

"Henry, I just met an interesting man, Mr. Underwood, the tall man over there, who . . . ."

(Next day)

"Mary, I met an accountant last night, Mr. John Underwood, who had some interesting ideas about investing money." (Writes name in address book.)

Moreover, she reinforces her use of the new name. She repeats the name back to him, uses it in addressing him, and then introduces and describes him to others. The reinforcement is immediate, placing the name in long-term memory, and then the memory path is exercised a few minutes later and again the following day. Again, "Use it five times and it's yours."

There are two other easy ways to minimize certain kinds of memory problems. Do you forget where you put things? Here, you have probably put the thing in so many different places over time that you don't have a good memory cue as to where it is. The key to this is to work on discipline and order. Simplify things, throw unneeded things out, have a regular location for things, and try to minimize disarray. "A place for everything, and everything in its place." When you can't do this, carry a note pad and jot down locations. "Parking lot—car three rows from the store on the right."

Do you forget to do something you were meaning to do? Here, the problem is not a memory problem as much as it is neglecting habits that you used well earlier in life. During our child-raising and working years, most of us as a matter of habit made lists. Lists for the grocery store, lists as to when to pick up the kids, reminders to ourselves about the hair appointment or the social engagement. Many seniors have simply gotten out of the habit. Carry a small daily diary and make lists of the things that you want to do. Cross them out after they're done.

Jogging the memory is simply a matter of exercising it. You need to work systematically to remember the unremembered things and to review the now-unfamiliar territory. As you redo your index, you bring a great variety of forgotten thoughts into your thinking process and reopen your mind to the richness of your past experience.

Exercising the Mind

The mind is a marvelous thing, but, like your body, it won't keep itself up unless you pay some attention to it. You need to exercise it. It helps if the exercise is the right kind for you. Much of our intellectual power is based on our memory and past experience. But a lot of other activity of the mind consists of actively acquiring *new* knowledge. Review your own activities, and see if you are doing enough mental exercise. Television game shows and police dramas are usually not terribly effective exercise for the mind, nor is reading the same viewpoint over and over again in slightly different form.

Variety and *challenge* are important attributes for new inputs. Variety means using many different sources—different newspapers, magazines, books, public television. Mix entertainment with serious content in a way that is comfortable to you. Reread old things to jog your memory and reestablish memory paths, but read new things too. Beware of "tabloid" sensationalist type inputs, because they may clutter your store of knowledge with inaccurate information.

Challenge means seeking out viewpoints that are opposite your own. Discussions with people who disagree with you can be much more stimulating (although perhaps sometimes uncomfortable), compared with discussions with people who think just as you do. Our contemporary world has a wealth of information sources and viewpoints. Seek them out. A good exercise is that of becoming, at least once in a while, "the devil's advocate." Marshal the arguments against your usual point of view; sometimes you will find that you have gotten an important new insight. Many of our daily activities, even the marginally unpleasant ones, are good mental training; and it may help a little bit to think of them this way. Balancing the checkbook and going over the income tax are a couple of examples. Pleasant activities exercise the mind as well. Crossword puzzles and card games such as bridge, concentration, or even poker are mental stimulants.

Problem-solving has been held to be the most central feature of human intelligence. While it is no particular fun to have problems, the solving of them can be satisfying or even exhilarating. And the subsequent freedom from the problem opens up other areas of your life.

Problem-solving activities, to be efficient, need to be systematic. Usually the problem and the approaches to its solution need to be written out. Planning a desired trip can be a problem. The alternative, not going on the trip, is usually an unfortunate choice of a solution. But you need to plan for travel arrangements, itineraries, things to wear, places to stay, friends to accompany, and myriad other details. Getting the car fixed can represent a whole series of difficulties, easily dealt with if you have a systematic plan but otherwise fraught with frustration. Compensating for problems with mobility caused by arthritis may represent a very complicated problem, and solutions may involve doctors, friends, exercise activities, compensatory activities, and many other factors. The very process of problem-solving keeps you alive in the fullest sense.

One important aspect of problem solving is represented by the important phrase "Always have a Plan B." You want not only to have a primary plan, but also a fall-back position. The primary plan is Plan A, and your alternative is Plan B. (Sometimes you need Plans C, D, and E.) A problem with problems is that they don't always have solutions. Or a particular solution, no matter how well planned, may not work in some instance. Without a Plan B, some of these unavoidable failures can develop into a frustrating feeling of helplessness and low self-esteem. There are always alternatives, and these need to be a part of your plan.

Fighting Depression

The greatest enemy to the healthy senior mind is depression. When you are depressed, everything slows down. You think and move more slowly. You have more difficulty solving problems. You are always on the verge of the vicious cycle of frustration and deeper unhappiness. Many seniors are depressed, and some are seriously so. The symptoms include not only "feeling blue," but also problems with sleep and with daily activities. Fortunately, there are very effective ways to manage all kinds of depression. Be active, be good to yourself, anticipate, plan, look forward.

Exercise is a marvelous antidepressant. It gets you out and around, releases endorphins in your brain, and improves your physical abilities. Mental exercises improve your cognitive abilities. Medications, on the other hand, tend to aggravate depression, often seriously. Nearly any drug can cause depression on occasion, and you should always discuss this possibility with your physician. Notoriously, codeine, sedatives, tranquilizers, and alcohol increase depression.

New activities and hobbies fight depression effectively. Voluntary and public service activities are extremely helpful. Humor is a very effective antidepressant. Medication in the form of antidepressant drugs can be extraordinarily helpful. We don't think that antidepressant drugs should be used first or for minor depression, since the natural approaches have their own rewards and are enough for most people. But depression can be serious and even life-threatening. Your feeling of depression should always be interpreted as a serious problem and one that needs discussion with your doctor. Depression is not an essential part of aging, and its negative influences need to be minimized.

Wisdom

Wisdom is the essence of mature intelligence. The attributes of age, including wide experience and a broader range of inputs than those available to the younger, make wisdom an attribute that you can cultivate as you age. Wisdom is an "inductive" process. It does not derive from taking a number of facts and deducing an exact solution. Rather, it takes a broad array of past experiences and new inputs and focuses them on solution of present problems. It is aided by having your memory organized, well-oiled, and frequently used, and at the same time incorporating new information into your wider perspective. You will have your own particular brand of wisdom and your own particular style of expressing it. Wisdom is the ultimate expression of your mature intellect.

CHAPTER 11

Senior Sexuality

The times they have changed. As we have matured, society has become much more open in sexual expression and discussion. Seniors can either benefit or suffer from the new freedom of sexual expression. The new freedom comes from recognition that active sexuality can be an important part of the later years. The anxiety comes from the ideas of sexuality of our youth. From this background it is sometimes difficult to adapt easily to new sexual attitudes. Sexual intimacy can continue to be a meaningful part of your life at any age.

Changes with Age

Whatever your age, the sex hormones are still released in the bloodstream in both men and women after stimulation, and they in turn stimulate the sexual organs. The sexual sequence, beginning with desire and progressing through orgasm to recovery, slows down but otherwise doesn't change much with age. Most people tend to continue the patterns of sexual expression that they had during their younger years. Those who were reserved and not particularly active sexually often find it quite easy to assume a more sedate sexual life and may not regret the lack of a sexual outlet. On the other hand, people who were more sexually active during mid-life and who derived great enjoyment from sex will probably continue to do so. If you have a suitable partner, you can continue to have an active sex life into your old age. In some ways, your physical needs and abilities may change, but you will learn to modify your sexual activities to fit your abilities. For many seniors, the sense of an emotional connection during sex is deeper in the later years. In later years, men need more foreplay and take a longer time to arousal, while many women tend to climax more quickly; often these changes can improve a sexual relationship.

The Woman

After menopause, some women feel that their sex life is mostly over. Pure myth. Freedom from the possibility of pregnancy sometimes makes sexual relations more relaxed and pleasurable. There are, however, declining levels of the female hormones, especially estrogen. As a result, most women notice a decrease in vaginal lubrication and a less elastic feeling in the vaginal wall. The lessened lubrication means that it can take longer to feel ready. Intercourse itself may feel rough, scratchy, or painful. The vaginal walls, with less estrogen, become thinner, and this can cause cracking, bleeding, and pain.

There are three ways to deal with the problem of lubrication. Frequent intercourse itself actually helps solve these problems. The vagina is stimulated to produce lubrication locally by intercourse itself. Second, estrogen therapy (such as Premarin) can help maintain the capability for vaginal lubrication by providing replacement estrogen. Since estrogen is also helpful in maintaining the strength of your bones and preventing osteoporosis, estrogen replacement therapy is something every woman should discuss with her doctor. Third, local lubricants can be used.

These can be estrogen or other creams applied to the vagina or use of a lubricant jelly (preferably water-based) immediately prior to intercourse.

Some women worry that hysterectomy, bladder suspension surgery, or other surgical operations have made sexual activity undesirable. Not so. Your reproductive organs (uterus and ovaries) have little to do with the physical or emotional aspects of sexual enjoyment. After removal of uterus or ovaries, you should be able to return to normal sexual activity. Similar problems sometimes arise after removal of a breast for breast cancer. Here the problem is even more obviously that of self-image. The best defense against judging yourself by superficial standards is to understand that your attractiveness is based far more on your inner-self than on your physical attributes. Sexual attractiveness, particularly for mature individuals, includes the values of character, intelligence, warmth, and intimacy.

The Man

In later life, men undergo physical changes in their sexual behavior. It takes longer to achieve an erection than it did. The angle of the erect penis is less. The rigidity is decreased. Some men fear that these delayed or partial erections are a sign of impotence. They are not. In the same way, many older men who have had surgery on their prostate gland think that they will no longer be able to be active sexually. Again, this is not accurate. It is unusual for prostate surgery to affect physical sexual abilities. Moreover, temporary or episodic impotence in elderly men is common. Indeed, all men are impotent on occasion throughout their lives.

The fear of performance failure can itself lead to lower performance. It is important to be able to discuss the situation and the fears with your partner so that you can learn together to slow down the pace a bit. It is important to be able to talk with your physician, since frequently help is available. Commonly, a medication being taken to reduce blood pressure may be affecting sexual function. Alcohol becomes increasingly a sexual depressant as you age. Common tranquilizers and sedatives can have the same effect. If you have had a heart attack, you may fear that sexual excitement may bring on another attack, and this fear may show itself as impotence. Sexual excitement should actually be good for heart disease. Even if you are having anginal chest pains during intercourse, there are frequently medical solutions. For example, your doctor may suggest nitroglycerin tablets taken before sexual intercourse.

Other frequent changes are a decrease in the amount of ejaculate, a shorter period of imminence just before orgasm, decreased force of ejaculation, and a requirement for a longer period between intercourse. These are to be expected and don't really represent much of a problem.

The Situation

If you have a long-term sexual partner, your problems with senior sexuality are likely to be relatively few and to have ready solutions. Touching, caressing, expressing affection verbally, hugging, and other forms of intimacy can be extremely satisfying. Even with illness of one or both partners, there are usually ways of expressing sexual intimacy that are mutually pleasurable. You may need to discuss needs and desires with your partner more specifically than you are used to, and this can be difficult. You may need to experiment a bit. You may need to deliberately schedule some time so that you can both come to the moment with anticipation.

If you do not have a permanent sexual partner, fulfilling sexual needs is more difficult. Women often have more difficulty finding appropriate partners than men, in part because they traditionally have not been expected to take the initiative and in part because older women are more numerous than older men. Fear of AIDS has become a social impediment to newly intimate relationships; for seniors this is not often a real problem, but the possibility does need some prior discussion between partners. Yet, some of the most touching and successful romances we know have occurred in later life. There is something wonderful about a new emotional and physical relationship that is not at all a monopoly of youth.

Masturbation can be a useful and satisfying way of achieving sexual satisfaction. Masturbation is acknowledged as a normal process of human sexuality. But many seniors have negative feelings for religious or personal reasons, and the teachings of the past may extend to the present. We don't recommend forcing any kind of sexual activity with which you are not completely comfortable just so that you can be "sexually active." Consider the whole range of possible options, but adopt only those with which you feel truly comfortable.

The essence of human sexuality is warmth and contact with others. Don't be afraid to hug your friends, your children, or your grandchildren socially. The physical parts of sex are electives, not requirements. Freedom from the sexual pressures that drove so many parts of our life when we were younger allows a greater range of choice. Greater available time permits deeper personal intimacies, whatever their sexual content. Recognize that the stereotype of old age as asexual, like other aspects of the aging stereotype, is wrong. But remember also that you don't have to prove anything anymore.

CHAPTER 12

The Healthy Home

Your home environment needs to fit you—your plants, your pictures, your bric-a-brac. You want the feeling to be comfortable and your personality and your tastes to be expressed in your surroundings. But your home can be your enemy in two ways. First, it can be sufficiently disorganized so that every activity of daily life becomes more difficult than need be. Second, your home itself can be dangerous. Many of the threats to your health come from your own home.

Ease and Routine: The Yearly Inventory

By organizing your surroundings for convenience, you create free time. It is axiomatic that time spent to organize is repaid many times over in time saved in daily activities. A more efficient routine gives you more time for other areas of your life that you want to develop. Solving unrecognized problems of your daily routine can allow initiation of new activities. A yearly inventory of your home is an important part of your plan for living well.

The main problem is clutter. It has been said that coat hangers multiply in the closet like rabbits. Medicine chests quickly fill to overflowing with outdated and dangerous nostrums. Unread magazines pile up on end tables. The last surviving glass from each old set of glassware collects dust in the back of the cupboard. The solution is in the discard. The ancient and honorable ritual of spring cleaning is a most rewarding custom. In our overfilled society, generally less is best.

At least once a year (and it doesn't have to be in the spring) throw out and reorganize. Usually it is best to break up this task into little sections, first because it is quite an effort and also because you can get absorbed in the life review as old objects trigger reminiscences as you sort through them.

From the medicine chest (or wherever you keep medications), get rid of all the outdated prescription bottles. It can be dangerous to take old medicines since they may have deteriorated in the bottle and represent a different chemical. Toss out all the free samples that came in the mail that you haven't used yet. See how empty you can get the cabinet. A good goal is to try to get down to a small tin of adhesive bandages and a bottle of acetaminophen tablets (Tylenol, Anacin) for minor pain syndromes. If you are living with someone else, be sure to keep your medications separate to avoid confusion. Don't exchange or share prescription medicines at any time; often there are reasons that certain drugs can't be taken by all people, and you may not know these reasons.

Go through the clothes in closets and dressers. A good rule is that if you haven't worn it in three years, you don't need it. By applying this rule, usually you will find that you have quite a pile of clothing that can be donated to a charitable organization, making it available to people less fortunate than you.

In the kitchen, the same rule applies: If you haven't used it in three years, you probably don't need it. It will be easier to find the things you do use if the clutter is reduced. While you're sorting through the kitchen, think about its overall organization. You want the things that you use most frequently to be easily accessible. You want them near the place (sink, stove, etc.) where they will be used. Don't be afraid to have duplicates of things you use a lot. You want heavy items to be in positions below shoulder height and above floor level.

Go through the garage, storage areas, or attic. These are filled with memorabilia and can be a wonderful place to spend a morning or a week. Here there are always many things that can be thrown out, but there are other things that are treasures of your past and that are important to keep. The broken lamp should clearly go, but that box of old pictures should perhaps be sorted, identified, labelled, and kept.

Someplace you have valuable documents (financial documents, wills, marriage licenses, passports, birth certificates, and so forth). When you are reorganizing, make sure that important documents are all kept together and that they are well labelled so that you (or others) can find them. Make sure that they are in a safe place, since some are irreplaceable and others are difficult to duplicate. If you are worried about safety of such documents, consider a safe deposit box at your bank. Often these are available free of charge to senior account holders.

Protection Against Injury: The Safety Inventory

Accidental deaths and injuries, almost by definition, are preventable. You do need to know the things that are most likely to cause trouble so that you can avoid them. As we age, the actual frequency of accidental events does not change too much, but the number of injuries and deaths that result are greatly increased since our bodies are less able to withstand injury.

Table 12–1 lists accidental death rates for different age groups. Note that while motor vehicle accidents are a continuing threat throughout adult life, for seniors they have been surpassed as a cause of death by falls and the resulting injuries. Deaths due to fire are also highest in older populations.

The automobile environment is your home away from home and needs to be healthy too. Here, the first essential is to always keep your seat belt buckled. This cuts your risk of motor vehicle death by about one-half. The second rule is not to be in an automobile when the driver is intoxicated or impaired. This will eliminate about half of the rest of the deaths. Additional guidelines are to drive within your abilities, to stay off the streets when possible at dangerous rush hours or late at night when problems from other drivers are greatest, and to be sure that visual and hearing aids are used when driving. A final tip is to discipline yourself to use the rear view mirror and the side mirrors regularly while you are driving.

Table 12–2 lists a brief safety inventory that may suggest possible improvements in your home environment. By paying advance attention to safety planning, you can substantially decrease the frequency of falls, other injuries, and fires. The basic approach to avoiding falls is not to have things around that you could trip over and to make sure that your common routes to and through the house are free of hazard. Loose throw rugs are a frequent cause of falls, as are slips getting in and out of the bathtub. If you're having trouble getting in and out

TABLE 12.1. *Accidental Death Rates (Number per 100,000 per year)*

Age	*Vehicle Accidents*	*Falls*	*Fires*
1– 4	7	1	4
5–14	7	1	1
15–24	36	1	1
25–44	20	1	1
45–64	15	4	2
Over 65	22	31	5

of the tub, be sure that there is nonskid tape on the floor of the shower or tub and that you have good handles available. Don't trust pulling on the soap dish. Tangled electrical cords across the floor can be a menace. Sharp corners can cause injury with even small falls. Rails and banisters need to be in good repair. Stairs should be free of debris, outside steps free of ice and snow.

If you are going to use step stools to reach high items, make sure that they are sufficiently stable for your ability. Often it is better to have someone else do the high tasks. If you have organized your house right, you shouldn't have to get things off the top shelves very often, but there are always burned-out light bulbs. A surprising number of falls come from inadequate foot wear; shoes should be practical, comfortable, and flat. Lighting should be adequate—another substantial number of falls come from not being able to use your vision adequately to protect your balance. A night light can often be very helpful.

If you don't smoke, your risk from fires and flames is already down by one-third. You can reduce it further by rehearsing how you would get out if there were a fire and by having inexpensive smoke alarms to give you early warning. Keep the fireplace well cleaned and use the screen when it is lighted. With your good diet, you won't be doing much deep-fat frying;

TABLE 12.2. *Safety Inventory*

Throw rugs	**Stairways**
Electrical cords	**Rails and banisters**
Night lights	**Step stools**
Sharp corners	**Ventilation**
Smoke alarms	**Fire exits**
Lighting	**Fire extinguishers**
Gas stoves and heaters	**Safety shoes**
	Door and window locks

this is good because flame-ups at the stove are another common cause of fires.

Work through your common routes about the house with particular care. Bed to bathroom. Living room to kitchen. Outside porch to living room and kitchen. Make sure these routes are clear of hazards.

Another frequent cause of falls is getting up a bit too fast. Many of us are subject to momentary dizzy spells as we rise quickly. From the bed, sit first, then rise. Stand a few seconds before leaving the bed so that your body blood vessel reflexes can adjust to your erect posture, and then proceed. Your exercise program helps protect against injury because it keeps your bones and muscles stronger; it both protects you against falls and decreases the chances of injury if you should fall.

Home safety is another example of how planning ahead can help you maintain good health. It also demonstrates how planning can help you compensate for physical problems you may have. Your techniques for avoiding injury are probably entirely different than when you were younger, but they can be just as effective. Falls are greater threats, football injuries less. In your car, you are less likely to run into things in front of you; you are more likely to be rear-ended.

Anticipate home problems *before* they occur. If I were to fall in or around the house, where would it most likely be? What is the greatest fire danger in my dwelling? What are my own greatest automobile hazards? What about security from break-ins? How could I call for help? Every situation is different, but the same commonsense principles operate. Recognize that in your home there are substantial threats to your health. Identify the most likely areas for problems, and then develop a plan to eliminate or reduce the hazards.

CHAPTER 13

Retirement*

Retirement gives you the opportunity to spend your time your way. It allows you to make changes you want to make. It greatly increases the flexibility and decreases the pressures of your life. On the other hand, retirement can represent boredom. It can seem as though the purpose of life has been lost. You can find yourself in relative isolation, and you can find yourself in relative poverty.

So much has been written about the problems and opportunities of retirement that it all seems very familiar. Some people thrive after retirement; some seem to begin to go downhill. Clearly, there are many different pathways and there is no single correct course for everyone. As a mature decision maker, you don't want to reject any options out of hand; you want to consider the entire range of available choices and then select the ones you prefer.

You may have already made your initial retirement decisions. Don't feel that these are in any way binding. You can change direction at any point. For the average individual, the period after age 65 is about 16 years long—for many it is 20 to 30 years.

*For help with the discussions of this chapter, I am particularly grateful to my most-senior reviewers, Albert Charles Fries and Orpha Hair Fries, who, in addition to making this book possible, have contributed the wisdom of octogenarian and septuagenarian to these pages.

This is far too long to represent a single phase of the life cycle; there is ample time for three or four different phases within "retirement."

Options

WORK OPTIONS

The *work option* continues to be available for many seniors. What you decide to do about it depends largely on how you feel about three things. First, how well did you like your old work, or how eagerly do you look forward to new work that you might undertake? If your work was unpleasant for you, this suggests that you may be better off not working. Second, are the other new activities that you plan to develop compatible with continuing to work? If you have alternative activities planned that have real appeal, this is another signal against the work option. Third, will additional money from working make much difference in the way you live? If not (and you will see from the rest of this chapter that it likely will not) this is another signal not to work and to more totally enjoy your new flexibility.

Within the work option are multiple suboptions. You can continue your past work activities after retirement age—you can delay retirement. Many self-employed people, in particular, like this option. Or you can take a new job, perhaps in some totally different area. You can phase down with part-time work or you can phase up by undertaking a new kind of part-time employment. The attractiveness of the various alternatives depends on individual preferences, the realities at the work site, and even the national economic cycle, so choices become very personal. We have seen very successful senior lives follow each of these several tracks. Again, no decision is a final one. You can reevaluate yearly. You should seriously reevaluate at least every five years.

ACTIVITY OPTIONS

The activity options of retirement provide even more alternatives. You can move or stay where you are presently living. You can go closer to the children or farther away. You can undertake entirely new hobbies or develop the old ones. You can travel or not. Again, your emphasis should be on conscious consideration of all the possibilities and careful, deliberate choice among them.

Make a list of all the things you might like to do. Be imaginative. Make a complete list, including the crazy possibilities, and then prune it down and select. We have no specific advice except for one general suggestion. Break with the old stereotypes of aging in at least some ways. When a choice comes between an active and a passive activity, choose the active. Do, don't sit. Many studies indicate that health and activity are closely interrelated.

LIVING OPTIONS

With the retirement period often 20 or more years in duration, you will need to reevaluate your living situation, and perhaps change it, several times. Generally, if you elect a new living option, you will be moving into smaller quarters with greater amounts of services provided for you. There are advantages and disadvantages to each choice, and both the choices you make and the timing with which you make the move are important to aging well.

Table 13–1 outlines just a few of the major options and lists some typical advantages and disadvantages. You need to make your own list and think it through, at least once every five years. In addition to the practical considerations, there are many less tangible ones that depend on you and the particular options available. Where are your friends? What is the local reputation of each facility? Will your choice encourage regular physical activity or discourage it? How highly do you value home ownership? Do you like upkeep chores or not? How do you project your physical function over the next five years? What is the age range of people with whom you would like to share experiences, and how does this compare with the age range

TABLE 13.1. *Living Options*

	Possible Advantages	*Possible Disadvantages*
Living at Home: Keep old house Move to condo/trade down Move to retirement community in Sun Belt Sell house and rent Continue to rent	Familiar surroundings Knowledge of community Near old friends and neighbors, church, etc. Costs possibly less Home health care paid mostly by Medicare	Medicare does not pay for any household help when needed If round-the-clock companion-aide is needed, difficult to get and keep desirable help Plumbing, house repair, etc. Dependence on neighbors, family
Shared Housing: With one other person With several	Companionship Exchange of skills Security Reduces cost	Compatibility: neatness vs. sloppiness, talkative vs. quiet, common interests or not Maintenance (painting, plumbing, etc.) Responsibilities for each must be clear
Retirement "Home"/ Hotel:	Companionship and shared activities Meals available in-house Maintenance provided Other services available, some at additional cost	No health care—only 24-hour "switchboard" One must move if he or she becomes chronically ill—these facilities are not licensed by state to give any hospital or medical care
Complete Retirement Home: Buy in Rent	Companionship and shared activities Meals planned in-house Entertainment as desired Planned transportation to symphony, museums, shopping, restaurants Health care—convalescent care Laundry, cleaning, and maintenance Opportunities for service	Cost, monthly Substantial investment Some have not been financially stable

of a particular facility? How much do you value being close to family? What are your financial resources? How much do you value guaranteed entrance into a long-term care facility?

Start with a blank page and make your own list of advantages and disadvantages. Then think over the list carefully. The "right answers" are likely to be different for different people. A basic principle is to make a choice that preserves options for future choices, that leaves you "in control." However, "independence" is itself a little different for everyone. For example, you can actually become more independent by electing a housing alternative that provides many services rather than staying in your own house if this choice increases your ability to do other things that you want to do.

NURSING HOMES

Institutional care in a long-term care facility is required at some point by about one-fourth of seniors. Some 6 percent of the over-65 population and 21 percent of the over-85 population live in such facilities. If you have a chronic disease, the chance that you will need long-term care at some point is greater than if you do not. There is a tendency for slightly older ages of admission to nursing homes over time as the senior population improves its average health status and as home care and other services increase in availability and diversity.

Here again the choices, both choice of facility and choice of timing, are often very individual ones. Nursing homes are frequently classified by the level of nursing support provided, from those with low-intensity care to those with highly skilled and specialized treatment. At any given level of service, there is a wide diversity among different facilities both in the quality of medical care and in the quality of life afforded.

Your research into the available options should precede the actual need for care. Enlist the help of family, friends, and your doctor in assessing alternatives. Make a list similar to Table 13–1 for the different possibilities. Consider finances, location, access for friends and family, access for your doctor, reputation, types and problems of other patients, further options if you later require more skilled help, presence or absence of waiting lists, criteria for admission, and any other factors that are important to you. Consider also the purchase of long-term care insurance. While there are major forces encouraging national long-term care insurance programs, these do not yet exist, and at present you need to check your coverages and make your own provisions.

Finances

Money problems are often more soluble than you think. Seniors as a group are more affluent than any age group except that of 45 to 64 years. Moreover, necessary expenses are generally lower than at any other period of adult life. Taxes are usually less. Of course, there is an extremely wide range of individual situations. Many seniors are on fixed income without assets, and their financial flexibility is limited. Many more seniors have substantial (but often hidden) resources; these resources are often "hidden" in nonliquid assets such as house and land.

Today's seniors are extremely conservative in fiscal matters. This is a result, in part, of having lived through the Great Depression, in part by having developed the habit of gradually accumulating assets by hard work, and in part by value issues such as worry about being a burden to others, particularly to the family.

Some of the reasons for financial conservatism are based on stereotypes and should be carefully reexamined. As a first principle, you should consider all your hard-earned money your own. It doesn't belong to anybody else. After establishing a suitable reserve, you should consider a plan to spend it all. In this day and age, at the time of your death your children are beginning to approach retirement themselves. They shouldn't need your money, and if they do, it isn't likely to change their lives very much. If your own financial examination shows you to be in extraordinarily good financial health and you have more money than you need for the rest of your life, you should consider giving it away *during* your life. Support of children, grandchildren, universities, or charities can be very satisfying, and you are in a much better position to see that your wishes are carried out when you are still around to check up.

THE FINANCIAL EXAMINATION

You should conduct a brief examination of your financial health every year. With this knowledge, you can then construct a financial plan and either continue the present plan or change as is appropriate. We strongly recommend that you do not perform this process entirely by yourself. If you have any assets at all, you need a trusted financial advisor, whether it is a professional, a friend, or a family member. Be very careful in your choice of someone to confide in since, if they lead you to bad decisions, there obviously can be bad consequences.

The essential part of your yearly financial examination is to estimate your personal "net worth." This is a simple task, although it is often made to seem complicated. Basically, you just need to answer the questions represented by the first seven lines of Table 13–2. Skip all the small and hard-to-figure things such as the value of miscellaneous items, furnishings, or the car. Then follow the seven steps. (1) Estimate your house equity, which is its present estimated market value minus any outstanding loans you have on it. (2) Estimate the cash value (not the face value) of any life insurance that you have. (3) Estimate values of any stocks and (4) any bonds that you hold. (5) List in round numbers any savings that you have, including savings accounts, savings bonds, certificates of deposit, and other monies kept in banks. (6) If you own any additional real estate, estimate its value minus any outstanding loans. (7) If you have any other major assets, put them on the final line. If you have any major indebtedness, put it in with a minus sign.

Add these numbers up and put the sum on line 8; this represents your approximate net worth. The size of the total will surprise most people. A typical senior, exemplified by column II of Table 13–2, will have approximately $100,000. Almost everyone who owns his or her own house will fall roughly in this category. And in those areas of the country where the typical person is less well off than this, the rents and house prices are generally more affordable. Depending on the area of the country, 10 to 25 percent of seniors fall in the excellent situation outlined in column I (or even a better one). On the other hand, depending on whose figures you use, as many as 25 percent of seniors fall into the fixed income without assets category represented by column III.

TABLE 13.2. *Finding Some Extra Money*

	You	*I—Excellent Situation*	*II—Typical Situation*	*III—Fixed Income*
1. House (value minus loan)	_____	**$150,000**	**$ 75,000**	—
2. Life insurance cash value	_____	**20,000**	—	—
3. Stocks	_____	**10,000**	—	—
4. Bonds	_____	—	—	—
5. Savings	_____	**25,000**	**25,000**	**$10,000**
6. Other real estate	_____	**50,000**	—	—
7. Other	_____	_____	_____	_____
8. ESTIMATED NET WORTH (add lines 1–7)	_____	**$255,000**	**$100,000**	**$10,000**
9. Reserve Fund	_____	**$ 25,000**	**$ 20,000**	**$10,000**
10. Available assets (line 8 minus line 9)	_____	**$230,000**	**$ 80,000**	**0**
11. Number of years needed	_____	**23**	**15**	
12. Available capital per year (line 10 divided by line 11)	_____	**$ 10,000**	**$ 5,300**	
13. Available interest per year (6% of line 10)	_____	**$ 15,000**	**$ 6,000**	
14. Total extra cash per year (line 12 plus line 13)	_____	**$ 25,000**	**$ 11,300**	
15. Total extra cash per month (line 14 divided by line 12)	_____	**$ 2,100**	**$ 900**	

FIGURING YOUR AVAILABLE EXTRA INCOME

This discussion doesn't take into account your fixed income from Social Security and pensions. It deals with the calculation of *extra* money available to you from other sources. The arithmetic has been simplified for purposes of illustration. *The basic point is that you can spend about 1 percent of your estimated net worth every single month for a very very very long time, perhaps a quarter of a century, while still maintaining a good reserve.* The reason for this is that even as you spend your hard-earned money, the money you have not yet spent continues to make money for you by interest or by appreciation of assets.

To see how this works for you, fill out lines 9 to 15 of Table 13–2. First, (9) establish the amount of your assets that you want to keep as a minimum reserve. If you have a minimum amount that you want to leave in your will to others, put it in here. (If the reserve needs are larger than your estimated net worth, then you can't continue the exercise. Subtract your reserve from your net worth to see if this is the case.) (10) Otherwise, continue by choosing the number of years for which you would like extra income. Look up your life expectancy in Table 1–1 in Chapter 1. Most people should add five years to this number to stay on the conservative side. On the other hand, if you have a known medical condition that decreases your life expectancy, you may wish to choose a shorter number of years. Put the number of years on line 11. Couples should usually estimate longevity by the wife's figure.

Divide your available assets by the number of years. This gives you line 12, the available capital you have to spend each year. To this you can add line 13, the interest you will receive each year. For convenience, assume an average interest rate of 6 percent per year for all your assets. This includes appreciation of a house or property, as well as interest on various financial assets. This is a conservative rate.

Add the available capital to the available interest, and you have line 14, the total extra cash available to you each year. Divide this number by 12 and you have the total extra cash (extra because it doesn't include Social Security, pensions, and other income) available to you each month. Three examples, for people with greatly differing financial resources, are shown in columns I, II, and III.

Column I represents Tom and Betty Jones, a recently retired middle-class couple both presently aged 66. Their suburban house, bought in 1955 for $50,000, is now worth $180,000, and they have an outstanding mortgage of $30,000; thus their house equity is $150,000. Tom has a paid-up life insurance policy with a face value of $20,000 and thus a cash value of $20,000. Betty has some stocks that she inherited a few years ago, currently valued at $10,000. The couple has $25,000 in savings, carefully accumulated over the years, mostly in two certificates of deposit of $10,000 drawing 7 and 8 percent interest. The Jones have a half interest in a lake house that they share with friends; they have had this property share for nearly 20 years, and their equity is approximately $50,000.

The estimated net worth of this middle-class retired couple is over a quarter of a million dollars. They would like to set a minimum financial reserve of $25,000, leaving them $230,000 in assets. On the other hand, their life expectancy is great. Betty's life expectancy at age 66 is about 18 years—adding 5 years for safety gives them a 23-year pay-themselves period.

Thus they have about $10,000 of available capital per future year for nearly a quarter of a century. In addition, their assets, assuming a conservative 6 percent per year, are increasing at a rate of slightly over $15,000 per year. So they can safely spend an additional $25,000 per year in addition to their fixed income, or about $2,100 per month! These simple calculations should be approximately accurate for five years, at which point Tom and Betty should recalculate—the new figure will have a little less interest income but not much.

Mary Smith, a 77-year old widow, has considerably fewer assets, as shown in Column 2. Her modest home, valued at $75,000, had the mortgage retired 10 years ago. She has been living on her fixed income from Social Security and survivor benefits from her husband's pension and has hoarded $25,000 in savings against a rainy day.

Mary's net worth is $100,000. Setting aside $20,000 as a minimum reserve, she has $80,000 in available assets. Her life expectancy is about 10 years, and adding 5 years gives her 15 years to use for financial planning purposes. This gives her about $5,300 of available capital to spend each year, to which she can add $6,000 in interest for a total of $11,300 per year, or about $900 per month. Using this money will more than double her monthly budget!

Scenario III is not as positive. Without equity in property and with only a small savings reserve, Florence Doe, a 71-year-old widow, must, to be prudent, essentially live on her fixed income. There are some things she needs to be sure to do, but we will discuss them later.

Note that the couple in Column I are financially independent for life. With pension and Social Security, they have $4,000 a month to spend, very low taxes, and a very low mortgage payment. Yet they may well have thought they were financially strapped.

Mary Smith, the elderly widow represented by Column II, is also in quite a comfortable financial situation. She has available to her nearly $1,000 a month in extra funds for the rest of her life.

This kind of calculation should be repeated each year, or at least each five years. Very gradually, the portion available from interest will decline; on the other hand, if interest and appreciation average more than 6 percent, net worth may stay close to the same or even go up.

LIQUEFYING ASSETS

There are some practical problems that come between Tom and Betty Jones, Mary Smith, or yourself having all these assets and realizing the income from them. These problems center around the differences between *liquid assets* like savings and the relatively *fixed assets* represented by your house and other property. To use funds from your liquid assets is easy. You just transfer the predetermined amount to your checking account each month; often this can be done automatically by the bank. Assets such as life insurance can either be cashed in and the money invested in liquid savings or you can take a series of loans against the cash value. Usually it is best to make regular transfers each month into your checking account, although some people like to do it in bigger amounts when there is a particular need.

The problem is with the fixed assets tied up in property. Here, there are many things that you can do. Most likely, you will want to keep your emergency reserve in the house equity. You are probably never going to need this reserve and so it doesn't need to be very accessible; should you ever need it, you could then sell the house. If you have extra property, it can be placed on the market and sold at an appropriate time and the cash transferred to the stocks, bonds, or savings lines of Table 13–2. Generally, we don't recommend selling the house in any big hurry since it is both a major part of your life and usually an excellent investment. But sometimes a house has just become too much for you and you would like to sell it. Then you just invest the proceeds as you want among the stocks, bonds, and savings lines of Table 13–2. Note that nothing really happens to your total estimated net worth (line 8) or to your ultimate financial plans when you move funds around from one line to another. You haven't spent anything; you have just rearranged your assets.

"Trading down" is a good option for many people. Sell the house and buy a smaller house or condominium. Invest the profit. Currently, profit on the house is tax-free up to $125,000. (You can only use the tax exemption after age 55, and you can use it only once.) This tax break is designed to help seniors trade down without financial penalty, and it can help you liquefy your assets. Suppose that you bought your house many years ago for $40,000, the mortgage is paid off, and it is now worth $210,000. Subtracting the $10,000 you have spent on improvements, you have a net profit of $160,000. If you now buy a condominium at $90,000, the difference of $70,000 is not taxable (once). You will realize $210,000 minus $90,000, or $120,000 to invest. Moreover, you will have less upkeep to worry about.

Table 13–3 lists some other strategies for liquefying capital from your house. The "reverse mortgage" is frequently heralded as the solution to the cash flow problems of seniors, but, surprisingly, these mortgages haven't yet caught on and are often not available. Ask if your bank offers reverse mortgages and check out the terms carefully. The American Association of Retired Persons has excellent materials available to explain these mortgages (see Appendix C, "For Further Reading"). Unfortunately, some banks are using "reverse mortgage" to charge interest rates of 20 percent or more; avoid situations with unreasonably high interest rates, even if they are hidden by the lender requiring a share in future home appreciation.

You can use a home equity credit line just like a second mortgage. Second mortgages are readily available, and you also can use them like a reverse mortgage. Second mortgages may cost a little more or a little less depending on the interest that you get for the mortgage money that you invest elsewhere and the interest costs of the second mortgage. With tax savings and careful investing, this technique can sometimes work out better than the others. The key is what the effective rate is: Look for the lowest. Using the second mortgage technique, you borrow an amount, say $50,000, against your house and then invest the money in a liquid investment and pay yourself from this investment each month.

All these different options come out about the same financially. For example, assume that you have a house worth

TABLE 13.3. *Options for Liquefying Your Home Equity*

Trading down	**New first mortgages**
Reverse mortgages	**Home equity credit lines**
Second mortgages	**Selling the house**

$130,000, with a first mortgage of $30,000, giving a home equity of $100,000. You can either take out a reverse mortgage, acquire a home equity credit line, or take out a second mortgage for $50,000. Assume an interest rate of 12 percent to make the calculations easy. You want to withdraw $1,000 a month. With the reverse mortgage (or the home equity credit line), the first month you get the whole $1,000, but the second month you have to pay interest on $1,000, the third month interest on $2,000, the fourth month interest on $3,000, and so forth. Your interest costs, therefore, slowly rise at $10 each month.

On the other hand, at a home appreciation rate of 6 percent per year, your house is silently appreciating $650 every month. For a second mortgage example, assume that your investment returns 9 percent, whereas you are paying 12 percent for the mortgage. (If you can decrease this "spread" this option looks even better.) Under current law you will have a substantial interest income tax deduction. With these assumptions, your interest payments the first month are $125 and thereafter increase by $7.50 each month as you gradually spend the money. Note that there are some disadvantages in having a house "free and clear." It is not a bad idea to stay borrowed (up to 80 percent of the value of the property) since this increases your "leverage" for appreciation of the value of the house and provides the greatest amount of tax advantage.

Let's see how things look after four years. Appreciating at 6 percent a year, the house now is worth $164,000, whereas the first mortgage has decreased to $25,000. After subtracting four years of paying yourself $1,000 a month ($48,000) the net house worth is about $90,000. After four years of taking $48,000 out, your equity in the house has only gone down by $9,000! You still have over nine-tenths of that equity left. Moreover, the house appreciation each month has now gone up to $820. Your financial situation with the different alternatives is almost the same. Interest expense is getting to be a sizable cost, but on the other hand the rate of house appreciation has been rising too.

Looking at the other basic alternative, which is to sell the house, the numbers don't come out very differently. When you sell the house, we assume that you net $100,000 and invest it at 9 percent. You take $1,000 a month from these investments for additional cash. Your nest egg, however, makes $750 each month, so you only have to dip into the capital at an initial rate of $250 a month. Even after five years, you will still have $86,000 or so left in the nest egg, will still make substantial amounts of interest from it, and have only slightly increased the amount that you have to dip into the capital each month to maintain the $1,000 a month. You don't have additional interest costs per month as you did with the mortgage alternatives, but you now do have to pay some rent, so it all comes out about the same. If you keep your house now but sell it after three years, seven, or even ten the numbers work out similarly.

You can spend up to 1 percent of your assets every single month for a very, very long time; not 100 months as you might first think (although even this is over eight years), but actually for perhaps 300 months. You can spend some of your assets and have them too.

AVOIDING LOSS

Each year thousands of seniors are the victims of swindles that rob them of their savings. Those swindles, such as the "pigeon drop," usually play on your sympathies, less often on appeals to greed. For the most part, you can easily avoid these swindles. *Never* invest with strangers. *Never* take a lot of money out of the bank without talking it over with your trusted financial advisor. Report any suspicious conversations to the police—you may help others.

The quality of the investment advice you receive is critically important. The technique described above for liquefying capital and very slowly spending down your assets is extremely conservative, as long as your investments are prudent. You should never gamble with your assets. Almost always, you should invest for "income" rather than "growth." You should not make risky investments. There are many sound, conservative investments including savings bonds, certificates of deposit, broad-based income stock funds, broad-based income-oriented bond funds, and others. Except in unusual circumstances, you should not change your investments more than once every several years. Changing investments costs money. If an unscrupulous investment advisor "churns your account" by frequently changing the investments, the financial advisor's commissions rise and at the same time your account balance decreases.

WHEN ASSETS ARE LOW

Suppose that your situation is represented most closely by scenario III, in which you are in fact limited to a fixed income without any assets that you can convert into monthly cash. Here, your situation unfortunately doesn't allow as much flexibility, and you need to work on the "expense" side of your budget rather than on the "income" side. You will have to increase your living standard by being frugal. If you have a car, it may well be worth getting rid of it and its total cost of perhaps $2,000 per year. Shared housing with a friend or with family might be appropriate. If you are frugal with the big costs of housing, food, medical care, and transportation, the smaller items tend to take care of themselves.

Worrying too much about "being a burden" if things turn bad can increase problems. You supported your children for 18 years or more when they were growing up, and they can support you now. Fair is fair. Besides, if you are successful in breaking the old stereotypes, who says you have to be a burden? You can be a help. Families with more members can distribute the needed tasks more efficiently. Baby-sitting the grandchildren, running errands, or even just waiting for the repairperson to come can be positive contributions. Too frequently we hear public commentary about how elders shouldn't live with their children, but on the other hand we bemoan the breakup of the "nuclear family." The active elder can be an asset and not a burden.

Then, too, there are many ways for seniors to save money that are not generally available to the rest of the population. Subsidized housing, subsidized public transportation, and discounted restaurant meals are just a few examples. Taxes are lower, and Medicare takes care of a good chunk of medical expenses. The American Association of Retired Persons and magazines such as *Modern Maturity* frequently discuss hundreds of ways in which your expenses can be reduced.

Retirement is better when you have financial flexibility as well as time flexibility. For most people, a conservative plan to gradually reduce assets can result in important infusions of income and thereby provide this increased financial flexibility. For others, limited to a fixed income, the emphasis has to be on limiting expenses. In all cases, you benefit from a plan, some good personal advice, and from exercising your whole range of choices. Aging well includes maintaining your financial health too.

CHAPTER 14

Completing the Plan: *Advance Directives*

You want to stay in charge of what is done to your body even if you someday become powerless to directly affect it. You want to be able to distribute your financial assets in the way that you choose. These desires require some planning and some decision making. You need to formally execute "advance directives" by which you specify in advance, formally and legally, what you want to happen. You have both personal health reasons and financial reasons for preparing advance directives.

National polls consistently show that over 80 percent of our population desires a dignified death, without artificial life support in the terminal situation. The overwhelming majority of us do not wish to die on tubes and respirators and among strangers. Yet fewer than 10 percent of the population have taken the appropriate steps to ensure that their terminal illness will be handled in the way that they want.

Eighteen percent of your lifetime medical costs, on average, will occur in the last year of your life, and most of these will occur in the last month. This represents in excess of $20,000 worth of health care services. These catastrophic costs can seriously deplete your estate, can cause financial hardship on your family, and form a significant part of the steady increase in health care costs and health insurance costs.

Why do so few people prepare adequately for their future? There seem to be two basic reasons. First, it is unavoidably an unpleasant task. You have to sit down and think about your death or incapacity and specifically make choices as to what you would like to have happen when you are seriously ill, dying, or dead. It is easy to procrastinate with a task like this. After all, you might die suddenly and not need any of this preparation anyway. And perhaps it seems like the problem is a long way away, and there is plenty of time to take care of these things later. The second reason is that the process of preparing advance directives is complicated and difficult to understand. The legal technology is obscure. If an attorney is involved, it may involve unknown expenses.

Actually, at most there are four advance directives you need: the living will, the durable power of attorney for health care, the durable power of attorney for financial/asset management, and your last will and testament.

There are obvious problems with attempting to give you specific recommendations here. The laws tend to be different in every state. Laws are changing every year, generally in a beneficial direction. Thus, more and more states recognize living wills, allow durable powers of attorney, and have simplified the process so that it is easier to understand. If the process is oversimplified, however, documents might not be legally binding, and you might not understand all the alternatives that are available. These legal procedures are intended to help you be confident that your wishes will be carried out, and you have many many options for expressing your personal wishes.

In the simplified discussion which follows, I have used a number of sources, including *The Power of Attorney Book*, by Denis Clifford (Nolo Press, 950 Parker Street, Berkeley, CA 94710, second edition, April 1988 [$17.95]). Even this book, written by an experienced attorney, warns appropriately on its title page:

> The information in this book changes rapidly and is subject to differing interpretations. It is up to you to check it thor-

> oughly before relying on it. Neither the author nor publisher of this book makes any guarantees regarding the outcome of the uses to which this material is put.

That disclaimer is clearly appropriate for the reader of this chapter as well!

Even Clifford's book, which is written for the general public, is complex and a bit intimidating. There are 19 different tear-out forms, each several pages in length (although you probably only need 3 of them). Different states often require slightly different forms. We have reproduced four of these forms and placed them in Appendix A. My recommendation is that you fill out these forms *if you agree with the basic assumptions of this chapter*. (The assumptions are summarized in Table 14–1.) If you want to execute the forms entirely by yourself, I recommend that you purchase *The Power of Attorney Book* and read all the appropriate sections. If you don't use that book, take the completed forms to your attorney when you are making out a will or reviewing your will, and thus obtain professional consultation before executing them.

Some people won't agree with the assumptions listed in Table 14–1. Perhaps you would prefer that everything possible be done to preserve your life for as long as medically possible under any circumstances whatsoever. This is your choice, and

TABLE 14.1. *Assumptions of this Chapter*

For the Living Will:
You do not wish your life to be artificially prolonged if you are terminally ill.

For the Durable Power of Attorney for Health Care:
You have a trusted friend or relative whom you would prefer to make medical decisions for you in the event that you are incapacitated, but not before.

For the Durable Power of Attorney for Asset Management:
You have a trusted friend or relative whom you would like to make financial decisions for you in the event that you are incapacitated, but not before.

For the Last Will and Testament:
You would like to personally specify distribution of your assets and simplify legal proceedings after your death.

under these circumstances, you certainly don't need a living will. Perhaps you don't have anybody who is close enough to you and whom you trust enough to be your agent for health care. Perhaps you don't have anyone whom you trust enough to manage your financial affairs without supervision if you are incapacitated. In that case, you may wish to fall back on the judicial process (which will appoint such a person in the event it becomes legally necessary). Although the process is more cumbersome and costly than a power of attorney, it offers numerous safeguards that can sometimes be worth the cost and the red tape.

This chapter assumes that you want to prepare advance directives, and that a major reason for you to prepare these is to ensure that extraordinary medical measures are not taken during your terminal illness. With these assumptions, the purposes of the four documents required can be easily understood. The functions of the documents are summarized in Table 14–2.

Don't procrastinate. Just starting the process of preparing advance directives is helpful. Even documents that are not legally "airtight" are of great use. For example, suppose that you had filled out and signed a form, had it witnessed by one person rather than two, didn't have it notarized, and were using the wrong form for the state in which you live. The docu-

TABLE 14.2. *Advance Directives: Your Final Documents*

The Living Will:
An advance directive that you do not wish your life to be artificially prolonged.

The Springing Durable Power of Attorney for Health Care:
An advance directive that specifies an agent to make medical decisions for you when you cannot make them yourself.

The Springing Durable Power of Attorney for Financial Asset Management:
An advance directive that specifies an agent to make financial decisions for you when you cannot.

The Last Will and Testament:
An advance directive for distribution of your assets after your death and for disposition of your remains.

ment will express your wishes, but it will not be legally perfect. It can still help, though, because you have made your wishes known. If you have given copies to your doctor and to the agent whom you have selected and to other members of your family, you have made your wishes known to others.

Consider the immediate benefits of preparing advance directives. Your doctor has a wide latitude in deciding how vigorous to be in managing terminal illness. Knowledge of your wishes can importantly guide these decisions. Some additional advice: Talk with your doctor about his or her philosophy of managing terminal illness. Doctors vary a great deal in their personal approaches, some wanting to do everything possible to preserve life for the longest possible time and others being concerned with painless and gentle death with dignity. You want your philosophy and that of your doctor to be the same.

As a second example, knowledge of your wishes will help your family make decisions that are consistent with your wishes. All too often I have seen a dying patient around whom the family converges from far away. The son who hasn't seen his mother, now in a coma, for ten years suddenly feels guilty and starts insisting that the doctor do everything that is humanly possible to prolong life. The doctor, who will generally be sympathetic to the family's wishes for a comatose patient, is placed in a difficult position.

Obviously, it is better to have the right forms, to have two witnesses, to have the forms notarized, and to have had the forms executed within the last five years. But just having made the initial effort will be of help.

The Living Will

The living will is the easy form to prepare. You don't need a lawyer. This is a directive to your physicians to avoid the use of life-support equipment. At least 39 states have adopted some form of living will law at the time of this writing.

The states with living will statutes (as of 1988) are: Alabama, Alaska, Arizona, Arkansas, California, Colorado, Connecticut, Delaware, District of Columbia, Florida, Georgia, Hawaii, Idaho, Illinois, Indiana, Iowa, Kansas, Louisiana, Maine, Maryland, Mississippi, Missouri, Montana, Nevada, New Hampshire, New Mexico, North Carolina, Oklahoma, Oregon, South Carolina, Tennessee, Texas, Utah, Vermont, Virginia, Washington, West Virginia, Wisconsin, Wyoming.

Living wills were the initial legal device used to deal with the ethical problems raised by the invention of life-support systems. Generally, the same form will work in all states, and even if a state does not have a living will statute, the document is still useful for the reasons given above.

The living will is not nearly as powerful a document as the "durable power of attorney for health care" discussed below, as it is addressed only to physicians and deals only with life-support systems. In many states it is not a legally binding document unless you are terminally ill when you sign it. However, we recommend that everyone who does not want life-support systems to be used in the terminal situation to read and complete the living will, to have it witnessed by two individuals who are themselves in good health, and that copies be distributed to physicians, family, and to one or two close friends. We recommend further that you repeat this process each five years so that a reasonably current document is available if it is needed.

The Durable Power of Attorney for Health Care

You need to understand the terms in the title "durable power of attorney for health care." "Power of attorney" means that you are granting someone else the power to act in your place.

"Durable" means that the power of attorney is active when you are incapacitated; ordinary powers of attorney are automatically terminated if you become incapacitated. "Health care," of course, means that this durable power of attorney is limited to health care decisions. In contrast to the living will, a power of attorney for health care is a legally binding document.

In many states you can use the same document to establish a durable power of attorney for health care and asset management, but in some states, such as California, you cannot. In any event, I believe it is better to think of these two durable power of attorney documents separately and to prepare them as separate documents, regardless of what state you live in.

Another term that you need to know is "springing." A springing durable power of attorney for health care becomes effective only *after* you are incapacitated. Until that time, you have not delegated any power to anyone. This chapter assumes that you will want a springing durable power of attorney. (The most frequent exception to this assumption is if you are already close to incapacitated and would like to delegate authority effective immediately.)

The durable power of attorney is a very powerful legal document. The document itself must contain strong warnings that you are giving away broad powers to your agent (termed your "attorney-in-fact"). If you retype any of these forms, you have to be sure that all the warnings are typewritten in capital letters.

Two forms of springing durable power of attorney for health care are provided in Appendix A, one for California and one for other states. Complete the appropriate form and have it witnessed and notarized. Be sure to talk with the person whom you have designated as your agent (attorney-in-fact) before formally executing the document. Again, we recommend that you either review your alternatives in detail through *The Power of Attorney Book* or that you consult with your lawyer. Since most people will want to talk with a lawyer about their will anyway, that lawyer visit is a good time to review all the advance planning documents.

The Durable Power of Attorney for Financial/Asset Management

With this document, too, you want your power of attorney to be "durable" so that it remains effective even though you are incapacitated. Indeed, this is when you want it to work. So again you almost certainly want it to be "springing," springing into action at the time at which you become incapacitated. In the terms of the form in Appendix A, determination of your incapacity must be made in writing by a licensed physician and you specify whom you would like the physician to be, if possible. You then designate your agent, or attorney-in-fact. If you want, you can appoint a second agent in case the first agent is unavailable or incapacitated him/herself. You limit the total authority of the attorney-in-fact by specifying that the attorney-in-fact cannot use your property for his or her own benefit, and you add a clause excusing any third party (such as banks) from responsibility if they were to mistakenly rely on a power of attorney that had been, for example, revoked. This clause helps ensure that the authority of your agent (attorney-in-fact) will actually be accepted in significant financial or property exchanges.

Again, you need two witnesses, notarization, and to repeat the process every five years to be sure that a current document is available when and if it is needed.

The Last Will and Testament

Everybody needs a will and everybody should look at it at least every five years to make sure it is consistent with current desires and appropriate for your current assets.

If you don't have a will, it causes a big nuisance for your survivors, and the legal expenses may eat up a good part of the assets. If your heirs start fighting among themselves, the whole business can get very sticky and expensive. If you don't have many assets, then you can use do-it-yourself will forms that are available in books on wills found at any good book store, but if your finances are at all complicated, it is worth your purchase of a lawyer's time. A considerable number of law suits are caused by doing it yourself and doing it wrong. Ask yourself if any possible beneficiaries might be likely to challenge the will; if so, it is a clear signal to use an attorney.

Be flexible in your thinking when it comes to deciding what you want to do with your assets. All too often people automatically leave their assets to be equally divided among the children. This may be perfectly appropriate for you, but again, it may not. As I pointed out earlier, your children are likely to be well into middle age before you die. It is relatively unlikely that the proceeds from your estate will make a major change in their lives at that point. You might consider skipping a generation and distributing the funds equally among the grandchildren. This is likely to result in a lower tax bite, and perhaps the money will arrive where it is more urgently needed. Or perhaps not. You have to decide.

Look at the options in Table 14–3. Waiting to distribute your assets until after you are dead is in some ways a very unsatisfying alternative; it is only one of three major alternatives. First (as we indicated earlier in Chapter 13), it is your money,

TABLE 14.3. *Your Options in Asset Management*

1. **Spend it all yourself.**
2. **Give it away while you are alive to:**
   A. **Family**
   B. **Charitable causes or institutions**
   C. **Charitable trusts for income.**
3. **Leave it for disposition in your will.**

and you are fully entitled to spend it all yourself. You can use the funds to increase your own standard of living for the rest of your life, even though this will decrease the value of your estate after you die. Generally speaking, you can spend 1 percent of your assets each month and never run out of money.

If you were planning on giving your assets away after you were dead, consider the possible advantages of giving them away while you are still alive. You can give to family, to friends, or to charitable institutions. If you are giving to a charitable institution, you can direct the use of the money more effectively while you are alive. Indeed, an institution that has received a gift is usually very attentive to your desires, in part because of the hope of receiving additional gifts. Perhaps you would like to provide a scholarship for a particular kind of student. Perhaps you would like to see some of your money go to protect the environment. Perhaps you would like to help a grandchild through college. If you have substantial assets, these are good ways to use them.

There is another possibility to consider. If you have substantial fixed assets (such as appreciated real estate) but are in need of day-to-day income, there is a way to be both altruistic with regard to charity and to protect your own income at the same time. Rules vary from place to place, but most universities or other large institutions that receive many gifts have offices that can advise you on the possibilities of "charitable trusts." These work something like this. You donate 100 acres of land to the university. The university sells the land and establishes a trust fund. The university pays you income from that fund for as long as you live. Thus, if the land were worth $1,000 an acre, the university would invest $100,000 for you, and if the fund made 10 percent a year you would receive $10,000 each year for as long as you live. You receive an income tax deduction in the year of your gift (based on the "actuarial value" or the projected "remainder interest" at your death. Upon your death, the money in the trust fund belongs to the university. Warning: There are various types of charitable trusts. The particular income tax consequences vary according to the type of trust and your own income tax situation. You should always discuss such a gift with your own income tax advisor.

Finally, in your will, whatever shape it takes, be sure to include your wishes with regard to funeral services, burial or cremation, and whether you want flowers or donations to some particular cause.

The Easy Way Out

This book is written for people with a wide variety of financial resources, from rich to poor. Partly for this reason, this chapter has emphasized do-it-yourself approaches to developing the advance directives that you need. To do this right requires quite a bit of effort.

The easy way out is just to make an appointment with a lawyer and tell him or her that you want to make or review a will, establish durable powers of attorney for financial/asset management and for health care, and to sign a living will. Typically this might take an hour in which you and your agent (attorney-in-fact) visit with the lawyer about your desires, a period in which the lawyer draws up the documents, a period in which the documents are mailed to you for review, and then a second session with the lawyer to go over anything that you don't understand and any changes that you want to make. If your assets are in any way substantial, say over $50,000, this time with the lawyer is likely to be a good use of your money. And once you have made that phone call to set up the appointment you have stopped procrastinating.

If you use a lawyer, fill in the forms in Appendix A first and take them with you. Just by filling them out you will have thought about most of the major decisions you have to make. This can save a good deal of time (and money) at the lawyer's office. It also will help that you are familiar with the documents that you need and with some of the terminology.

Completing the Plan

The basic message of this chapter is that almost everyone should want to prepare advance directives so that their wishes will be carried out through illness, terminal illness, and after death. The documents are needed now, and are an integral part of your plan for aging well.

CHAPTER 15

Surviving Chronic Illness with Style: Secondary Prevention

Most illness in the senior life stage is chronic. Chronic illnesses, such as atherosclerosis, osteoarthritis, emphysema, cirrhosis, diabetes, and the tendency to develop cancers, are conditions that may last for the rest of your life once you have them. The best approach to these diseases is to postpone them. This is called "primary prevention." In primary prevention, disease symptoms are postponed until later in life or even postponed so long that they don't happen at all during your life span. I have been talking about primary prevention in chapters 2, 3, 4, and 7.

There is another kind of disease prevention, however, termed "*secondary prevention.*" If symptoms from a disease are already present, your goal becomes to prevent the disease from getting worse. You now would like to prevent the disease process from causing very much trouble. Having failed in a *primary* sense to keep the disease from occurring, you now try a *secondary* way to prevent the disease from causing problems that can be lessened.

Often the same measures that are useful in primary prevention also act to slow the progression of a disease after it has occurred and, hence, are good measures for secondary prevention. This is particularly true with atherosclerosis. After you have had a heart attack or stroke or developed some other complication of atherosclerosis, it is particularly important that you implement the necessary lifestyle changes in addition to appropriate medical treatment. You already know that you are at high risk for another and possibly more serious episode, and it is extremely important that you work to prevent this. The principles of Chapter 7 apply to secondary prevention of atherosclerosis: a slowly graded exercise program, often under professional supervision; a diet low in total fat and saturated fat, stopping cigarette smoking; treating high blood pressure; and reducing weight.

With cancer, secondary prevention is also sometimes of help. Suppose that a skin or lung cancer was successfully removed or that a malignant polyp was removed from your colon. You know that you are at high risk for the same thing happening again. Hence there is an imperative for stopping cigarette smoking in the case of lung cancer, for attention to the appropriate dietary measures in the case of the early colon cancer, and for use of sunscreens after skin cancer.

One of the neglected principles of managing chronic illness is to isolate the chronic illness problems in a strong body. Exercise, both physical and mental, strengthens your entire body and minimizes the impact of the chronic disease. Increased attention to the prevention of other chronic diseases is also appropriate secondary prevention. It is much harder to compensate for the problems of two chronic diseases at the same time than for the problems of one. So, it is vitally important that you keep your general primary prevention program going even though you do have to contend with a specific problem.

Coping and Compensation

The term "coping" carries some negative connotations. When we say we have to cope with chronic illness it seems almost as though we are saying that we have to endure the pain and suffering. "Compensation" is a more positive way to view the process of adaptation to your chronic illness. You compensate by finding ways to do an activity more easily or to avoid the necessity of doing the hard-to-perform activity. You select an alternative activity that you can perform competently. The term "secondary prevention" is a little dry but means the same thing. You can prevent disability for a particular task either by improving your ability or by making the task easier.

We all need to cope with some aspects of aging. There are some things we can't do as we used to, and we have to adjust our activities and expectations accordingly. When we have a chronic disease associated with the aging process, it adds to this challenge. We may well have to develop alternative activities and to compensate. If you have major problems with stairs, you may need a ground-floor apartment or one with an elevator. If you have trouble with certain kinds of errands, you may have to arrange some home delivery mechanism. If you have trouble reading, you may need brighter lighting or stronger reading glasses. If red wine now upsets your stomach, you need to develop a taste for an alternative beverage.

As you select your alternatives, remember the mature coping mechanisms that are associated with good physical and mental health. You react with humor, with altruism, and with optimism. Everyone has some problems—you have yours. Some aspects of your situation will always be a little funny, and it helps if you can laugh at yourself a bit from time to time. Things can always be better than they are if you keep searching for improved alternatives.

We have discussed primary prevention in chapters 2, 3, and 4, and the specifics of making appropriate lifestyle changes in Chapter 7. These sections should be carefully reread by persons with chronic illness, from the perspective of their own personal problems. Everything in these sections will not apply, but most of it will. In the following pages, we discuss five common chronic disease processes in which secondary prevention is important: arthritis, osteoporosis, high blood pressure, diabetes, and Alzheimer's disease.

Arthritis

There are 117 different varieties of arthritis. For the most part, however, when we are talking about what older individuals call arthritis, we mean "osteoarthritis," also called "osteoarthrosis" or "degenerative joint disease." Most commonly, this kind of arthritis comes on very slowly and frequently involves the hands, the neck, the back, the knees, or the hips. The joint cartilage slowly wears away so that the inner surface of the joints becomes rough and irregular, and this can cause pain and loss of function.

However, much of what we call arthritis or rheumatism isn't caused by this roughening of the inner surface of the joints or the bony spurs that result. Rather, it is part of a complicated process that involves some arthritis and some muscular stiffness and soreness around the joints. Doctors have wondered for many years why people who have significant complaints and problems often have nearly normal joints on x-ray, whereas people who have very seriously affected joints on x-ray often function perfectly normally without any discomfort. The answer is that "rheumatism" is a complex problem involving a number of tissues, not just the joints. The tendency to develop this problem and for it to get worse increases with age. Depression, lack of exercise, and lack of pleasurable social activities make the symptoms worse.

There are three basic principles for primary prevention of osteoarthritis and musculoskeletal disability. First, keep fit. Exercise increases the strength of the bones and the stability of the supporting ligaments and tendons. Exercise nourishes the joint cartilage by bringing nutrients to the cartilage and removing waste products. Regular, gently graded, permanent exercise programs are required. Stretching exercises loosen up the stiffness in the joint areas and increase the range of pain-free motion in the joint.

Second, control your weight. Being overweight places unnecessary stress on joints by changing the angles at which the ligaments attach to the bone as well as by the additional impact on the feet, ankles, knees, hips, and lower back.

Third, protect your joints. Listen to the pain messages that your body sends, and perform activities in the least stressful way. Joints, ligaments, and tendons can be damaged by misuse of a part that is already injured. If you are suffering with discomfort from an activity, don't take pain pills just so that you can continue the activity. Listen to the pain message and change the activity appropriately.

Secondary prevention of the problems of arthritis involves these same three principles, but now this is only a beginning. You do want good exercise habits, for all the reasons discussed earlier. They will also retard the progression of your arthritis. You do need to control your weight—many symptoms of arthritis decrease or disappear entirely when you are at normal body weight. And you need to listen to the pain message that is coming from parts of your body that are injured and need rest.

Moreover, you may need medical help. If arthritis has become the major limiting factor in your life, we recommend that you see a rheumatologist (a doctor who specializes in joint diseases) for specific advice and guidance. If your problems are less severe, your primary physician can help, or you may very well be able to take care of them yourself.

Basically, you want to use medication reluctantly for osteoarthritis. Unlike rheumatoid arthritis and some other inflammatory kinds of rheumatic disease in which medication is extremely important, the currently available medicines for osteoarthritis are only symptomatic. They don't do anything basic for the disease and they may even mask some pain that might help you avoid further injury to the joints. There are serious side effects from arthritis medicines. Each year 2,000 or more people in the United States die from gastrointestinal (stomach) bleeding or perforation as a result of aspirin and other nonsteroidal anti-inflammatory drugs taken for treatment of arthritis.

This caution about drugs is not meant to be too negative. For many people these medications can be dramatically helpful, but if they don't seem to make too much difference for you, you may be better off without them. If you are having side effects, you need to trade off the discomfort and risk of side effects against the degree of symptomatic relief that you are getting. The major drug side effects are on the stomach, and many doctors and drug companies are working on ways to decrease this problem. Over the next few years, there will be some less toxic arthritis drugs on the market; there will probably be more use of acetaminophen (Tylenol, Anacin), which is harmless to the stomach; and some new drugs called prostaglandins may be available to help protect the stomach in addition to the antacids and sucralfates that are already available. Note that the acid antagonists, like cimetidine, do not appear to be protective.

With significant osteoarthritis, an important aspect of compensation is to take an inventory of your immediate environment. Ramps, rails, hard upright chairs rather than deep easy chairs, fat-handled utensils, canes, nonskid plates, and hundreds of other aids are available to make daily activities easier for individuals who have problems with them. We have detailed many of these in the *Arthritis Helpbook*, which has been written for the Arthritis Self-Management courses developed at Stanford University and now offered by the Arthritis Foundation. Scientific studies show that the Arthritis Self-Management course is about as effective as most of the medications available for osteoarthritis, and results in very substantial improvement. My book *Arthritis: A Comprehensive Guide* provides a great deal of background information on the different kinds of arthritis and what you can do to decrease problems. Complete information about these books is located at the back of this volume in Appendix C.

There is a major principle for dealing with all chronic disease, and it is particularly applicable to arthritis. *Take the long view*. Make choices that will result in your best function and your least pain over a substantial period of time—say two, five, or ten years from now. Short-term solutions (for example, painkillers, injections) sometimes may result in harm over the longer term. Thus you need to be a bit positive about pain, stiffness, and discomfort: they are major nuisances, but they are not the true enemy. What you want to prevent is disability, being unable to function as you would like.

Finally, a note about surgery. When severe osteoarthritis has destroyed a joint so that pain is continual and severe and function is impaired, surgery is frequently needed. Joint surgery has dramatically improved in recent years. Probably you know of several people who have had total hip replacements or total knee replacements. These joint replacement operations are now very commonly performed by many competent surgeons. They usually result in nearly complete relief of pain and in recovery of much lost function. Results are dramatic and immediate.

Just knowing that these good surgical procedures are available makes many people feel a lot better about their arthritis. The exact timing of surgery is not too important. When the problem from the arthritis has developed to the point at which it outweighs the risk, discomfort, and expense of the surgery, it is time to operate. The only caution is that you should not wait until your disability has become so severe that your muscles in the affected area have become weak and your tendons shortened, since then it is harder to recover full function after surgery.

Osteoporosis

It may seem as though almost everyone you know is "suffering from osteoporosis," yet osteoporosis by itself is not really a disease and doesn't cause suffering. In this condition, the bones have gradually lost much of their calcium. They have become weaker and more brittle, but they do not hurt! You can't "suffer" from osteoporosis; indeed, you can't even tell that you have it.

There is a tendency for all of us to lose calcium from our bones as we get older, particularly if we are not active. Exercise (particularly weight-bearing exercise like walking) acts to keep the bones strong. Hormones such as cortisone or prednisone can cause a much more rapid loss of calcium. Women tend to lose calcium more rapidly than men, particularly after menopause. Some diseases, such as rheumatoid arthritis, also cause loss of calcium.

While osteoporosis is not a disease, it can lead to serious problems with broken bones. These are what hurt. The vertebrae in the back can fracture (collapse) and cause much discomfort. A minor fall can result in a fracture of hip or wrist that would not have occurred if the bones were of normal strength. Fracture of the hip is particularly serious, but almost any bone can break.

Primary prevention, discussed earlier in Chapter 4, involves weight-bearing exercise, adequate calcium in the diet, and consideration of estrogen replacement therapy for women.

Secondary prevention begins when your attention is first focused on your osteoporosis because a bone is broken. Perhaps you were just going downstairs and suddenly felt a sharp pain in your mid-back that radiated around the sides of your trunk. Often a collapsed spinal vertebrae occurs without any major accident. This is a signal that your total body calcium has slipped down below the "fracture threshold," and that your bones are generally brittle. Remember that the calcium blood test that is frequently done has nothing to do with the amount of calcium in your bones. There are now x-ray procedures (osteodensitometry, CT scan) for measuring the amount of calcium in your bones, but these are not routinely needed. If something has broken rather easily, it is safe to assume that the calcium content of your bones is low.

After a fracture of the spine, as with other fractures, the healing process has to take place. This generally takes six to eight weeks. There is no good way to splint fractures of the spine, so you are going to have substantial discomfort. Generally, bed rest is not in your long-term interest, since this increases the loss of calcium from your other bones, which is the opposite of what you want to accomplish.

The secondary prevention principles for osteoporosis are the same as those of primary prevention. Women who have had osteoporotic fractures should very seriously consider estrogen therapy and should usually keep on with such therapy if they are already on it. Weight-bearing exercise should be gradually increased. Calcium intake should be at least 1500 mg per day.

The new thinking about bone calcium is that it is possible to return mineral to the bones and to do this relatively rapidly. The old thinking was that osteoporosis was a one-way street, and the process of calcium loss could be slowed down but not reversed. Now it is recognized that with careful attention to managing the risk factors you can slowly regain bone calcium. Don't expect this to be rapid, since it may well take two years just to get your bone strength back up above the fracture threshold, and you may never get back to your original bone density levels. But if you can get above the fracture threshold, you will be relatively protected against recurrence of this kind of problem. Repeating the principles: Weight-bearing exercise for all. Calcium for all. Estrogens for women. Decrease in prednisone or other corticosteroid drugs (if you are taking these and cutting down is medically possible.) Avoidance of falls. These are the principles, and if you follow them, you can save a lot of misery.

High Blood Pressure

High blood pressure (hypertension) is a uniquely silent disease. Many people who have high blood pressure do not know it. There are no symptoms until the high blood pressure has resulted in harm to the arteries. The catastrophe of a heart attack or stroke is all too often the first indication of a problem. You can't wait for headaches or nosebleeds to give you fair warning; these are not reliable indicators of high blood pressure. Actually, even if you do have these symptoms it is quite unlikely that they are due to high blood pressure.

Because high blood pressure is a silent disease process that can be treated effectively, early detection is important.

Primary prevention has to do with maintaining your body weight at a reasonable level, practicing aerobic exercise, not smoking cigarettes, managing stressful situations, and watching the salt in your diet. By these measures, many people can avoid the elevation of blood pressure in the first place.

Secondary prevention is needed after the blood pressure is found to be elevated. Here, the same measures that are effective in primary prevention can often return the blood pressure to the normal range and keep it there without medication. Remember that complications of high blood pressure come from the number of years that you have had it and the severity of the blood pressure elevation. These two factors combine to create damage to the arteries.

There is no emergency with mild blood pressure elevations. Indeed, we worry sometimes that the labelling of someone as "hypertensive" may make a perfectly healthy individual feel that he or she is sick. This is not a disease; it is a risk factor. If you attend to the risk factor, you can eliminate its contribution to future disease complications.

Importantly, there are many people with "high blood pressure" who don't need to be treated at all. Medical thinking has changed slightly in recent years so that we are now less aggressive in treating mild forms of high blood pressure. There are several reasons for this. First, many people's blood pressure is only up when they are in the doctor's office. Second, older people may need a little higher pressure to get the right blood flow through stiffer arteries. Third, there are side effects with the medications.

You need to understand a little bit about how your blood pressure is generated. The power comes from the heart. When the heart beats, it pumps blood under pressure into the arteries. Then the heart rests in between beats. You might think that the blood pressure would drop to zero at that point, but it doesn't. Instead, a valve at the heart snaps shut, preventing the blood from going back into the heart, and the elastic stretch of the walls of the arteries continues to pump the blood along. When the heart beats, blood is forced along, but the arteries are also stretched under the higher pressure. When the heart rests, the arterial walls constrict elastically and the blood is pushed farther along. The higher number of the blood pressure (systolic blood pressure) represents the strongest force of the heart beat. The lower number (diastolic blood pressure) represents the lower pressure while the arterial walls constrict. It is the lower number, the diastolic blood pressure, that is most closely associated with development of atherosclerotic plaques on the inside of the arteries and the complications of high blood pressure.

As you age, the walls of the arteries become less elastic. Thus, the heart needs to pump at a little higher pressure in order to maintain the flow throughout the heart cycle. It is all right,then, to have a somewhat higher systolic blood pressure as you get older. It doesn't need treatment. In younger individuals we rather arbitrarily define a normal blood pressure as one below 140/90. As you get older, a normal blood pressure might be 150/90, 160/90, or 170/90. This is why you sometimes hear that your blood pressure should be less than "100 plus your age."

If your diastolic (lower) blood pressure is over 105, you should be treated medically. Between 90 and 105, the situation is less clear. For most people in this range, restriction of salt, reduction of weight, reduction of alcohol intake, and exercise will help reduce blood pressure. Even keeping adequate calcium and potassium in your diet will help a point or two. (See Table 15–1 for the amount of improvement various home treatment methods can achieve.)

A further complication comes because blood pressure as measured in the doctor's office is not really the information we want to use for medical decisions. We really want to know your baseline blood pressure over the typical day. Many people have blood pressures that fluctuate up and down all the time, and this doesn't appear to be very harmful. Often this takes the form of "white coat hypertension," in which your blood pressure is highest when you are in the doctor's office. Obviously this can lead to your getting treatment that you don't need. Before you start treatment, you should have your blood pressure taken enough times and in enough places that you are sure that it is truly elevated. Get a blood pressure cuff designed for home use, learn how to use it, take readings frequently, and write down the numbers. This will help you and your doctor determine if you need treatment.

Another reason to be conservative with medication use is the side affects of medications. Blood pressure medications can make you dizzy, upset your stomach, or have substantial effects on your sexual potency.

Finally, if you do take medications, be sure that you are persistent and regular with your regimen. Many studies show that people with high blood pressure, because they don't have any symptoms, tend to take their medicine only some of the time. If you do require a blood pressure medication, take it exactly as directed so that you and your doctor can determine the right drug or drugs and the right dosage. If you have side effects, tell your doctor.

A frequently neglected treatment of high blood pressure is to treat your other cardiovascular risk factors. High blood pressure by itself isn't really a disease but a risk factor; it causes

TABLE 15.1. *Home Treatment of Hypertension*

Method	*Possible Decrease in Pressure*
Aerobic exercise	**5 points**
Maintain ideal weight	**1 point/10 pounds**
Low-salt diet	**2–10 points**
Adequate calcium intake	**2 points**
Adequate potassium intake	**2 points**
Relaxation techniques	**2 points**
Alcohol reduction	**1 point**

accelerated atherosclerosis. If you work hard on the other risk factors, you can minimize the chances of complications from the high blood pressure. So it is critically important to pursue your aerobic exercise program, your low-fat and low-cholesterol diet, and to avoid cigarette smoking.

Table 15–1 shows the effects of various forms of home treatment on the diastolic blood pressure. Typically, an aerobic exercise program can reduce the diastolic pressure by five points. Weight reduction achieves about a one-point reduction for every ten pounds that you lose. A low-salt diet helps some people a great deal, others much less. You get additional small improvements in blood pressure from having an adequate calcium intake and an adequate potassium intake. Stress reduction and relaxation techniques can be helpful as well. You can see that if you pursue all these approaches, mild hypertension can usually be adequately controlled without medication. Indeed, most people with high blood pressure probably don't need medical treatment. However, you do have to closely monitor the effectiveness of your home treatment program. Severe hypertension will not be adequately controlled by home treatment; mild hypertension can get worse with time. It is a good idea to have a blood pressure cuff at home. (Either get one that can be used with one hand or have someone help you take your blood pressure regularly.) We recommend making a graph or keeping a short diary to show how your blood pressure is doing. You can take your diary or graph with you to the doctor and discuss whether a medication change (either up or down) is required. Generally,

TABLE 15.2. *Prevention of Complications*

1. **Compliance with medication schedule**
2. **Home treatment program**
3. **Low-fat, low-cholesterol diet**
4. **Avoid cigarettes and other forms of nicotine**

if you can keep the diastolic pressure averaging in the 90 to 95 range or below, you are doing about as well as you can do. Table 15–2 reviews how to prevent the complications of high blood pressure; refer back to Chapter 7 for details.

Diabetes

Diabetes mellitus is a disease that occurs in two forms. The early-onset, insulin-requiring kind of diabetes is complicated and difficult to manage. You need a good doctor to work with you on this one.

By far the most common form of diabetes, however, is "maturity-onset," non/-insulin-dependent diabetes (NIDDM). As we grow older, our bodies become less able to handle a high sugar load. The sugar gets into the bloodstream, and the body is very slow in getting it from there into the body's cells. Thus the blood sugar levels remain high and excess sugar may be excreted in the urine, causing diabetes. This condition is one of "impaired glucose (sugar) tolerance." The normal changes in sugar metabolism with age merge with the disease syndrome of maturity-onset diabetes. Everyone has some trouble with glucose tolerance as they get older, and those who have the most trouble are defined as having diabetes.

This common kind of diabetes can usually be managed without medication, but not without a doctor. The two key treatments are weight reduction and aerobic exercise. Weight reduction itself can completely control diabetes in most individuals who are substantially overweight. Aerobic exercise, as we have discussed earlier, improves your metabolism so that glucose can get into the cells more effectively.

You will want to discuss with your doctor the other efforts that you can make to control your diabetes. Diet is very important, but "diabetic diets" are often confusing. The basic principle is easy. You want to avoid a heavy carbohydrate (sugar) load at any time during the day, because this is what your body is having trouble handling. If you spread your calories out into four meals, with a large breakfast, a large lunch, a smaller dinner, and a late-night snack, you avoid having too many calories come into your system at the same time. Thus, your body has more time to clear the sugars from the blood. Complex carbohydrates such as cereals and whole wheat grains are helpful since they release their sugars more slowly and more evenly, again giving the body more time to clear the sugar from the blood.

Complications of insulin-dependent, early-onset diabetes (typically beginning in childhood or young adult life) usually begin to appear after 15 or 20 years of illness and can be very severe. These involve problems with the retina in the back of the eye, problems with the kidney, problems with the nervous system, and accelerated disease of the vascular system. In the more common late-onset mild diabetes, these complications are more unusual.

The major problem in adult maturity–onset diabetes is acceleration of vascular disease; with your diabetes you have just picked up another risk factor. Hence it is critically important that you pay close attention to managing all your other cardiovascular risk factors. Your low-fat, low-cholesterol diet, control of high blood pressure, avoidance of cigarettes and other forms of nicotine, and moderation of salt are very important. These changes go along with your weight reduction and exercise program to help prevent complications. If you do have an early form of kidney disease, decreasing the protein in your diet may be effective in slowing progression and you should talk with your doctor about appropriate levels of dietary protein.

Alzheimer's Disease

The specter of Alzheimer's disease is one of the most fearful of all our anticipations of aging. Alzheimer's disease can end in senility. It is chronic, progressive, and degenerative. There is no cure and there is no good medical treatment. You have read many articles (and will read many more) about how the frequency of Alzheimer's disease is increasing rapidly in the United States. Sometimes you will see projections that in such and such a year some huge proportion of the population will suffer from this problem.

Alzheimer's disease is indeed a major national health problem, and it deserves both respect and commitment of a major national research effort toward its solution. But it is important to keep this disease in perspective. Fear of Alzheimer's can act like a disease too. While there is no really good news about Alzheimer's, there are some more positive perspectives that are rarely mentioned in the popular press.

First, relatively few people will get any form of Alzheimer's. Only about 5 percent of the population over 65 will ever have this problem; 95 percent will not.

Second, the only reason that we expect so many more cases of Alzheimer's in future years is that the population of older individuals is increasing. Your personal chances of getting Alzheimer's aren't very different from your parents' chances when they were your age. Over the past eight years, life expectancy figures from age 65 and from age 85 for women have been approximately constant and are likely to remain so. Since the trend toward living longer and longer has greatly slowed, the alarmist projections that are so commonly seen are exaggerated.

Third, many people with Alzheimer's only develop relatively minor symptoms. Because Alzheimer's disease comes on so late in life, many people will die of natural death or of other causes before the Alzheimer's has had time enough to become severe. Indeed, some of the changes that are seen in the brains of Alzheimer's patients are found as part of the normal aging process as well.

Fourth, of all the forms of senile dementia, Alzheimer's makes up only about half of the cases. Most of the rest is "multi-infarct dementia," which is felt to be cousin to atherosclerosis, and to be preventable in large part by control of the usual cardiovascular risk factors. No risk factors for Alzheimer's disease itself have yet been identified, although one study has suggested that cigarette smoking may predispose to later development of Alzheimer's.

Alzheimer's disease is difficult to diagnose early, because the symptoms, their severity, and the course of the disease itself vary greatly from patient to patient. A diagnosis generally is not made until the loss of intellectual abilities interferes with social activities.

Since there are no cures for Alzheimer's disease, treatment is partly focused on offering practical information for care givers—most often, close family members. Because Alzheimer's may cause stress within the family, both emotionally and financially, we urge care givers to seek psychological support and current information from friends, family, self-help groups, and professionals.

Remember that the momentary losses of memory that we all get are not a sign of Alzheimer's disease. We need to eliminate needless worry, anxiety, and attempts to hide or deny incidents of memory loss. Fear of Alzheimer's can itself become a phobia that impairs the quality of life.

For more information about Alzheimer's disease, you can contact the Alzheimer's Disease Society, 2 West 45th Street, Room 1703, New York, NY 10036, (212) 719–4744 for the chapter nearest you. You may also wish to read *Alzheimer's Disease: A Guide for Families* by Lenore S. Powell and Katie Courtice (Reading, Mass.: Addison-Wesley, 1982) and *The 36-Hour Day* by Nancy Mace and Peter Rabins (Baltimore, Md.: The Johns Hopkins University Press, 1981).

Chronic Conclusions

With chronic illness, your attitude toward the disease is as important a positive factor as the disease itself is a negative one. You need to stay in control. If you react with the feeling of helplessness leading to depression, you have coped unsuccessfully. The disease wins. If you take an active approach toward secondary prevention of complications and use coping mechanisms such as altruism, humor, and optimism, you can have a successful life despite chronic illness. An appropriate choice for many is to work personally toward solution of the disease problem in others as well as yourself. You can volunteer efforts to foundations and clinics working with the disease and you can contribute your personal efforts to the care of others.

If you make a long list of everything that you might possibly like to do over the rest of your life, chronic disease may make some of these difficult or impossible. On the other hand, you will find that there still is a long list of realistic alternatives upon which to focus your hopes and your efforts.

PART III

Solutions

Solutions

In this part, 45 common problems and their solutions are discussed. This section is for your reference. Look up your particular problems in the index or the table of contents or consult the list below. Then consult the appropriate pages to find your solutions.

Contents

Pain Solutions

Pain syndromes are very common, unpleasant, and a threat to the quality of life. Yet, pain is also a remarkably positive phenomenon. Pain is the premier defense mechanism of the body. Through it, you learn to avoid activities that can lead to long-term problems. Short-term pain is often your best protection against incurring damage that can cause more pain and dysfunction over the long term. Pain tells us to rest an injured body part until healing can be accomplished. Try to consider pain positively and learn to listen to its message.

On the other hand, pain can prevent activities or make activities uncomfortable, can encourage disuse, and can result in weakness of muscles and loss of bone calcium. There is a minor paradox here. If you heed the pain message too carefully, your functional abilities may atrophy. If you ignore the pain message, you may suffer long-term damage that will limit your activities.

There are solutions to this paradox. Respect the pain message. Analyze it. Reduce the effects of pain by natural techniques. Exercise the part in nonpainful ways, such as by use of isometric exercises. (These exercises alternately tense and relax muscle groups without movement.) Avoid medical pain killers, entirely if possible.

The following 16 sections provide specific natural solutions for different kinds of musculoskeletal pain and discomfort and provide a guide as to when to see the doctor for additional guidance and what to expect at the doctor's office.

1/ *Pain in the Muscles and Joints*

Pain in the muscles and joints is frequently termed "arthritis" by patients and sometimes by doctors, but most "arthritis" is not arthritis at all. The "arth" part of the word "arthritis" means "joint"—not muscle, tendon, ligament, or bone. The "itis" means "inflamed." Thus true arthritis affects the joints, and the joints are red, warm, swollen, and painful to move.

Arthritis is discussed as a general concern in Chapter 15. "Arthralgia" means pain without inflammation in the joints. "Myalgia" means pain in the muscles. These pains are *not* arthritis but can be very bothersome. Usually they are not serious and will go away. They can be caused by tension, virus infections, unusual exertion, automobile or other accidents, or can be without obvious cause. Only seldom do they indicate a serious disease. Rarely, thyroid disease, cancer, polymyositis (inflammation of the muscles), a disease termed "polymyalgia rheumatica," or other problems may cause arthralgias or myalgias.

There are over 100 types of arthritis and rheumatism. The four most common types are "osteoarthritis," "rheumatoid arthritis," "gout," and "ankylosing spondylitis." Osteoarthritis is usually not serious, occurs in later life, and frequently causes knobby swelling of the end joints of the fingers. Rheumatoid arthritis usually starts in middle or later life and may cause you to feel sick and stiff all over in addition to the joint problems. Gout occurs mostly in men, with sudden, severe attacks of pain and swelling usually in one joint at a time—frequently the big toe, the ankle, or the knee. Ankylosing spondylitis affects the back and joints of the lower back and may be suspected if your back is sore for a long time, particularly stiff in the morning, and you are unable to touch your toes.

Arthralgia and myalgia syndromes are much more common than true arthritis. Doctors often do not agree on diagnostic terms in this area, and two doctors may give different names to your problem. Some terms frequently used are "fibrositis," "nonarticular rheumatism," "psychogenic rheumatism," and others. Arthralgias and myalgias seldom progress to a serious condition. The consequences of arthritis occur very slowly and are often better prevented than corrected. Arthritis, arthralgia, and myalgia result in more lost work days due to sickness than any other category of disease.

Only rarely does a patient with arthritis or arthralgia need to be seen by a physician immediately. Home treatment will usually resolve the problem. The relative emergencies are (1) infection, (2) nerve damage, (3) fractures near a joint, and (4) gout. In the first three, serious damage may result if the joint is neglected; and in the fourth, the pain is so intense that immediate help is needed.

When to See the Doctor for Pain in the Muscles or Joints

- *Single, hot, swollen, painful joint without injury.*
- *Injured joint or other area not beginning to improve after four to seven days and preventing activity.*
- *Associated fever if not flulike, or if flulike, not improving after four to seven days.*
- *Associated weight loss or severe fatigue.*
- *Possible nerve damage with numbness, tingling, or pain radiating from the problem area.*
- *Persistence for more than six weeks despite home treatment.*

HOME TREATMENT

Both rest and exercise are important in treating muscle and joint pain. Try to relax and gently stretch the involved areas. Warm baths, massage, and stretching exercises should be used as frequently as possible. Sponge-soled shoes may help if you walk or stand on hard floors. Better light to help you relax a bit farther from the page or a better chair may help if you spend a lot of time at a desk. Regular exercise, slowly increased from very gentle to more vigorous, can help restore the proper muscle tone; we recommend walking, bicycling, and swimming. Aspirin, acetaminophen (Tylenol), or ibuprofen (Advil, Nuprin) are available over the counter and may be used in low to moderate doses. Specific techniques for specific types of pain are provided in the following sections. For more information, consult *Arthritis: A Comprehensive Guide* (by James F. Fries, M.D.), and *The Arthritis Helpbook* (Kate Lorig, R.N., Dr.Ph. and James F. Fries, M.D.)—listed in Appendix C.

WHAT TO EXPECT AT THE DOCTOR'S OFFICE

The physician will examine the joints, perhaps take several blood tests, and may x-ray involved areas. If a joint contains fluid, the fluid may also be removed and tested; this is not difficult or very painful. A cortisone-like drug may be injected (not more than three times) into a painful joint. Beware of the long-term oral use of drugs such as prednisone—their side effects may be worse than the arthritis. If drugs such as prednisone are to be continued for more than a few weeks, we recommend that a consultant concur in their use. In general, pain relievers containing narcotics or codeine are not useful.

2/ *Pain in the Lower Back*

Lower back pain is practically a universal problem. The crucial things to remember are that this problem is common (most people get it), painful (incredibly), medically minor (most of the time), and that the cause is nearly always an injury that requires time to heal completely. Medication cannot speed the healing process. If there is any sign of nerve damage, if a fracture might have occurred, or if it just won't go away, see the doctor. Sudden pain with minor or no injury occurring a bit higher in the back may represent a collapsed fracture of a vertebrae; this is the most common complication of osteoporosis and is a very frequent problem. This kind of fracture usually requires about six weeks to resolve, and many older persons will have several such fractures.

HOME TREATMENT

The purpose of treatment of acute low back pain is to prevent chronic, long-lasting low back pain. You want natural healing and then you want to strengthen the involved parts so that the problem doesn't happen again.

Think of these problems as similar to a sprained ankle, even though you cannot see what is actually happening. An injury causes bruising and swelling for two or three days, and then slow healing begins to become evident. The pain improves in less than a week, but six weeks is required for full healing. Reinjury is costly, since the healing process will have to start again from the beginning.

Do not take pain killers and muscle relaxants and then go on as if your back were all right; this practice has a high likelihood of resulting in reinjury. Either take medication and rest flat in bed, or listen to the pain message and do only what you can do in reasonable comfort.

Don't apply heat to the area the first day; if anything, use cold packs to decrease pain and swelling. Heat may be cautiously applied after the first day, but it won't help much. A firm mattress or a bed board is part of the standard advice; back problems vary, however, and if you are more comfortable at night and the following morning with a slightly softer mattress, use that. Aspirin or other mild pain relievers are probably all right, but they won't help too much. A small pillow or folded towel beneath the lower back may increase your comfort when sleeping flat. When you get up, draw your knees up, and then roll sideways and sit up. The position of lying on your side, knees up, is more comfortable than lying on the back for many people, and it is all right.

You doubtless have some accompanying muscle spasms. Although painful, they are protecting your injured back. If you can outlast the discomfort without muscle relaxants and without a lot of pain medication, your back may heal more strongly, and you decrease the chance of reinjury.

When to See the Doctor for Low Back Pain

- *Weakness or numbness in one or both legs.*
- *Pain going down a leg below the knee.*
- *Significant fall or possible injury.*
- *Fever without flulike aches.*
- *Persistence after six weeks of home treatment.*

Exercises shouldn't be started for a week or so, until things feel much better, and then they should be begun slowly. Exercise is designed to make recurrence less likely by toning the muscles and ligaments so that the spine has greater strength. Abdominal muscles assist spinal stability and are part of the exercise program. If you have some weight to lose, get started with the weight reduction right away.

Exercises should be repeated twice daily and gradually increased in number and in effort expended. Toe-touching, side-bending, and twisting exercises are *not* particularly good. For the back you are more interested in strength than in suppleness. Here are two good exercises: (1) Lie on the back and tighten the stomach muscles so that the hollow of the back is forced against the floor. Tense and hold for two seconds, relax, and repeat three times. Gradually work up to ten repetitions. (2) Lie on your back, pillow under your head. Hug your knees to your chest with your hands, exhale so that your spine can curve as much as possible, hold for five seconds, relax, and repeat three times. Work up to ten repetitions.

Good posture helps. Sit in a straight chair. Keep your shoulders back and down. Have a good mattress on your bed. Lift heavy objects using your legs, not your back. Never lift from a bending forward position. Avoid sudden shifts and strains, particularly those actions that throw the upper body backwards. Tennis, for example, should not be rushed as your back recovers. You can safely walk, swim, or bicycle long before it would be safe to resume an activity like tennis.

Adequate calcium in your diet is important to minimize the chance of fractures. If you don't have four servings a day of calcium-rich foods such as nonfat milk or low-fat ice cream, then calcium supplementation is advisable; this is very important for women. Women over 65 should have at least 1,500 mg of calcium daily and men at least 1,000. A glass of milk contains about 400 mg. The best supplementation is calcium carbonate, which is available as Tums or as Oscal or other similar brands. Women should discuss the pros and cons of estrogen supplementation with their doctors. Premarin and similar drugs can significantly reduce the chance of osteoporotic fractures.

WHAT TO EXPECT AT THE DOCTOR'S OFFICE

Unfortunately, don't expect too much. Unless there is nerve injury, the doctor does not have too much to offer. Surgery is best reserved for patients with nerve-compression syndromes or particularly severe and persistent difficulties. As most people know, failure of surgery to improve back problems is rather common.

The commonly used drug regimens of pain killers and muscle relaxants have never been shown to shorten the time of recovery or to help prevent recurrence; there is reason to suppose that under some circumstances these drugs can increase the chance of reinjury and can thereby delay healing. These drugs also affect your thinking processes and offer some hazard if you drive a car or operate heavy machinery. Uncomplicated low back strain is a problem for home treatment first. Similarly, massage, acupuncture, chiropractic, and other occasional treatments generally offer little that you can't do yourself.

If there is nerve injury, traction or surgery can help, and your delay in seeking medical care can have permanent consequences. So, keep looking for the danger signs of weakness, numbness, or pain going down the leg below the knee.

3/ *Pain in the Neck*

The neck bones are a continuation of the spine. The top seven vertebrae are called cervical or neck vertebrae. The seventh one makes the prominent bump that you can feel where your back joins your neck. The uppermost vertebrae, the Atlas, holds up the skull. The second vertebrae, the Axis, has a vertical peg (odontoid) around which the head turns. The entire neck is more flexible than the back; it bears less weight but is less well protected by thick muscles. The disc spaces in the neck can get narrow, bony spurs can form, and nerves can get caught and compressed, just as in the lower back. Arthritis such as spondylitis or rheumatoid arthritis can affect the neck, and rheumatoid arthritis is particularly likely to affect the top two vertebrae, allowing the head to slip forward and backward.

Excess tension in the neck muscles can cause neck pain as well and is probably the most common cause of neck pain. Here the pull on the ends of the ligaments causes pain in the back of the head where the neck attaches to the skull, and this pain can often shoot forward and be interpreted as a headache.

Usually, as in the lower back, a neck problem is minor and will be self-limited. However, injuries do take some time to heal. Healing depends on natural healing processes. Excessive neck movement tends to slow the healing and has the possibility of causing reinjury.

HOME TREATMENT

Rest the neck and listen for what the pain message tells you not to do. You can take a bath towel, fold it lengthwise so that it is a four-inch-wide strip, and wrap the neck with it, securing it comfortably with a safety pin or tape. Now you have a soft neck brace to wear at night, and this will clear up nearly half of all neck pain problems. If pain persists, use the soft collar during the day as well or buy a commercial soft collar to wear. You want some support from the collar, but more than that you want a little reminder not to turn your head too far or too fast.

Common sense says to watch out for things that aggravate the pain and to avoid them. Watching a tennis match is obviously not a good idea because of the repeated head turning required. You probably engage in other activities that require head turning and are just as damaging. For example, some people get help by wearing their glasses while reading because this enables them to be farther away from the book. Try to sit back farther from your work. Don't reach or look over your head to get objects; use a stool.

Keep pain killers and muscle relaxants to a minimum or avoid them altogether. Aspirin, acetaminophen, or ibuprofen are all right, but probably won't make you feel much better.

> ### When to See the Doctor for Neck Pain
>
> ■ *Numbness, tingling, or pain shooting up over the scalp.*
>
> ■ *Significant fall or possible injury.*
>
> ■ *Fever without flulike aches.*
>
> ■ *Weakness or numbness in the arms or legs, usually the arms.*
>
> ■ *Persistence after six weeks of home treatment.*

Sleep on a good firm mattress. Don't sleep on your stomach, and if you sleep on your side, place a pillow so that your neck is in a neutral position, not propped up or hanging down. When sleeping on your back, move the pillow beneath your neck as well as your head and keep the pillow a small one.

The time for exercise begins as the pain subsides, usually after five to seven days. Don't rush the exercises—they are designed to help prevent the next recurrence. There are two types of exercises, stretching exercises and strengthening exercises, and you should do some of each. Start stretching exercises with gentle stretches and increase the stretch slowly day by day. Do them twice daily, each maneuver three times gently. There are three maneuvers: chin toward chest, ear toward shoulder, and looking to the side. The last two should of course be done in each direction.

Strengthening exercises can begin at the same time and should start with three repetitions twice daily. Slowly work up to ten repetitions. If you have been having recurrent neck problems, these exercises are a worthwhile lifetime habit. Here are three: (1) Shoulder shrug—raise both shoulders toward ears, hold for two seconds, relax, repeat. (2) Take a deep, deep breath, hold for five seconds, release, repeat. The neck muscles are "accessory muscles of respiration" and breathing exercises involve the neck muscles. (3) While standing, grab one thumb with your other hand with both hands behind your back. Flex your head way back. Press down with your hand. Take a deep breath, relax, repeat. This exercise can be done lying on your stomach as well, after you get good at it standing up. A hot shower may increase comfort while exercising; some authorities recommend doing the exercises in the shower. (For safety hold onto something.)

WHAT TO EXPECT AT THE DOCTOR'S OFFICE

Uncomplicated neck pain problem is a job for home treatment first. If there is pressure on a nerve, then hospitalization, traction, myelograms, and surgery may be needed, but if there is no nerve pressure, the doctor has relatively little additional advice to offer. Surgery for the neck is sometimes hazardous and is inconsistent in relieving the problem. If your long-term neck problem doesn't have any "objective" findings and x-rays don't reveal a physical problem, the problem may be simply excess muscle tension. Tension headaches are a simple but bothersome problem that can localize in the neck muscles.

4/ *Pain in the Fingers*

Each hand has 14 finger joints, and each of these acts like a small hinge. Because the joints are small, they are operated by muscles in the forearm that control the joints by an intricate system of small slings for the tendon leaders. The small size and complicated arrangements mean that any inflammation or damage to the joint is likely to result in some stiffness and lost motion, as even a small scar or adhesion will limit motion. So, you shouldn't expect that a problem with a small finger joint will resolve completely. Even after healing is complete, some leftover stiffness and occasional twinges of discomfort are likely. Unrealistically high expectations lead to feelings that you did something wrong or that the doctor was no good. In fact, almost all of us have a few fingers that have been injured and remain a bit crooked or stiff. The hand functions very well with these minor deformities; fingers need not open fully or close completely to be perfectly functional.

Osteoarthritis frequently causes knobby swelling of the most distant joints of the fingers and also swelling of the middle joints. It can also cause problems at the base of the thumb. If we live long enough, all of us get these knobby swellings. They cause most of the changed appearance that we associate with the aging hand. Mostly, they cause relatively little pain or stiffness and don't need specific treatment other than exercise.

HOME TREATMENT

Listen to the pain message and avoid activities that cause or aggravate pain. Rest the finger joints so that they can heal, but use gentle stretching exercises to keep them limber and maintain motion. The key to managing finger problems is to use common sense.

With a bit of ingenuity, you can find a less-stressful way to do almost any activity that puts stress on the joints. Since everyone's activities are a bit different, you will have to invent some of these new ways yourself. Here are a few hints to get you going. A big handle can be gripped with less strain than a small handle, so wrapping pens, knives, and other similar objects with tape or putting a sponge rubber handle over the original handle can protect the grip. Lift smaller loads. Make more trips. Plan ahead rather than blundering through an activity. Let others open the car door for you. Get power steering or a very light car. Use a gripper for opening tough jar lids or stop buying products that come in hard-to-open jars. When opening a tough lid, apply friction pressure on the top of the lid with your palm and twist with your whole hand, not your grip. Cultivate ingenious friends who are handy at making little gadgets to help you. Don't put heavy objects too high or too low. Organize your kitchen, workshop, study, and bedroom.

When to See the Doctor for Finger Pain

- *Severe pain when fingers are at rest.*
- *Fingers cannot be straightened out.*
- *Significant injury.*
- *Numbness or tingling in the fingers.*
- *Persistence after six weeks of home treatment.*

Stretch the joints gently twice a day to maintain motion. Straighten the hand out against the table top. Make a fist and then cock the wrist to increase the stretch. Use one hand to move each finger of the other hand through from full flexion to straight out. Don't force, but stretch just to the edge of discomfort. If the motion of a joint is normal, one repetition is enough, but if the motion is limited, do up to ten repetitions. Warming the hands in warm water before stretching may help you get more motion.

Don't use strong pain medicines; they mask the pain so that you may overdo an activity or an exercise. Be sure that you take prescribed medication for inflammation just as instructed. Good hand function is important, and you want to pay close attention to treatment.

WHAT TO EXPECT AT THE DOCTOR'S OFFICE

The doctor will examine your hands and the finger motions. Sometimes a hand x-ray will be taken, but usually not more often than every two years. Antiinflammatory medications such as aspirin, acetaminophen, or ibuprofen can help, but doses should usually be low to moderate. Rarely, injection of a particularly bad finger joint is helpful, but this is less effective with small joints than with large ones. Surgery is also less effective with small joints and is not often indicated. Operations such as replacement with plastic joints or removal of inflamed tissue usually succeed in making the hand look more normal and may decrease pain, but the hand often doesn't work much better than it did before the operation.

5/ *Pain in the Wrists*

The wrist is an unusual joint because stiffness or even fusion causes relatively little difficulty, while if it is wobbly and unstable, this can pose real problems. The wrist provides the platform from which the fine motions of the fingers operate; it is essential that this platform be stable. The eight wrist bones form a rather crude joint that is very limited in motion compared with, for example, the shoulder, but which is strong and stable. Almost no regular human activities require the wrist to be bent all the way back or all the way forward, and the fingers don't operate as well when the wrist is fully flexed or fully extended.

The wrist platform works best when the wrist is bent upward just a little. To illustrate this position, make a fist and put your thumb in the middle of your fist. Looking down your arm, the thumb should be on an imaginary line going straight down the middle of your forearm. Thus, any item in your grasp, if the wrist is in proper position, can be pulled or pushed in the most efficient manner.

The wrist is very frequently involved in rheumatoid arthritis, and the side of the wrist by the thumb is very commonly involved in osteoarthritis. The carpel tunnel syndrome can cause pain at the wrist. In addition, this syndrome can cause pains to shoot down into the fingers or up into the forearm; usually there is a numb feeling in the fingers as if they were asleep. In this syndrome, the median nerve is trapped and squeezed as it passes through the fibrous carpel tunnel in the front of the wrist. Usually the squeezing results from too much inflammatory tissue. The cause can be tennis playing, a blow to the front of the wrist, canoe paddling, rheumatoid arthritis, or many other activities that repeatedly flex and extend the wrist. You can diagnose this syndrome pretty well yourself. The numbness in the fingers will not involve the little finger and often will not involve the half of the ring finger nearest the little finger. If you tap with a finger on the front of the wrist, you may get a sudden tingling in the fingers similar to the feeling of hitting your "funny bone." Tingling and pain in the carpel tunnel syndrome may be worse at night or when the wrists are cocked down.

HOME TREATMENT

The key to management of wrist pain is splinting. Since stability is essential and loss of motion is not as serious in the wrist as in other joints, the treatment strategy is a little different. Exercises to stretch the joint are not very important. The strategy is to rest the joint in the position of best function. Wrist splints are available at hospital supply stores and some drug stores. Any that fit you are probably all right. The splint will be of plastic or aluminum and the hand rest will cock your wrist back just a bit. You can put a cloth sleeve around the splint to make it more comfortable against your skin and wrap the splint on your arm gently with an elastic bandage to keep it in place. That's all there is to it. Wear

When to See the Doctor for Wrist Pain

- *Severe pain even when the wrist is at rest.*
- *Associated fever.*
- *Associated significant injury.*
- *Tingling in the fingers.*
- *Rapid development of swelling without injury.*
- *Persistence after six weeks of home treatment.*

it all the time for a few days, then just at night for a few weeks. This simple treatment is all that is required for most wrist flare-ups. Even the carpel tunnel syndrome is initially treated by splinting. But, since nerve damage is potentially serious, give your doctor a call if you seem to have the carpel tunnel syndrome.

No major pain medication should be necessary. Aspirin and similar-strength medications are all right but probably won't help too much. If you are taking a prescribed antiinflammatory drug, be certain that you are taking it just as directed; sometimes a flare-up is simply due to inadequate medication. If you know what triggered the pain, work out a way to avoid that activity. Common sense means listening to the pain message.

WHAT TO EXPECT AT THE DOCTOR'S OFFICE

The wrist will be examined and advice similar to that above will be given. X-rays may be required, but rarely. Antiinflammatory drugs may be prescribed. Injection with a steroid medication may be performed on occasion and is likely to be of help if a carpal tunnel syndrome has not responded to splinting. Surgery of several different kinds is available, and one or another procedure may be recommended in difficult cases. The carpal tunnel nerve compression may be surgically released. In rheumatoid arthritis, the synovial tissue on the back of the hand may be removed to protect the tendons that run through the inflamed area. The wrist may be casted or the bones fused.

6/ *Pain in the Elbows*

The elbow is really two closely related joints. One is a simple hinge joint that operates from straight to about 150 degrees of flexion. The second allows the forearm to twist. The first action allows us to eat, and the second is required to turn the soup spoon when eating soup. Several structures around the elbow may give trouble. Over the point of the elbow is the olecranon bursa sac, a frequent location for bursitis. On the inside and outside are bony bumps to which the muscles attach. These are frequent sites of tendonitis; for example, tennis elbow is a tendonitis on the outside bump of the elbow. The joint space can be the location of infection or even gout; these conditions will cause the part to hurt even when it is not being moved. The elbow is exposed enough so that fracture is not uncommon; this injury can be difficult to treat because the bones that usually break are right at the joint.

HOME TREATMENT

The basic treatment is rest combined with stretching exercises to prevent stiffness. If you know the cause of the problem, stop that activity. For example, a "tennis elbow" can be caused by a bad, jerky backhand that puts extra strain where the forearm muscle joins the bone. (You can get tennis elbow by using a screwdriver as well.) You can stop tennis or other activities for a while and you can later take some lessons to improve your backhand tennis swing. For tennis elbow (even when not due to tennis), an elastic strap over the upper forearm (available at tennis shops) will take some tension off the sore tendon.

Listen for the pain message and let it tell you what not to do. Avoid activities that either make it worse right away or increase pain on the next day. Remember that you have to let the inflammation subside and let the part heal. At least six weeks are required to build full strength. To avoid reinjury, your elbow activity must be below the level that would tear the weakened tendon fibers again.

Avoid strong pain killers, as they get in the way of your reception of the pain message. Aspirin, ibuprofen, or acetaminophen are all right, but they probably won't help you too much.

Take it easy with the elbow. The sling (triangular cravat) described in the next section on shoulder pain is the best way to rest it. Wear the sling all day for at least a few days; it will rest the elbow and will keep you from using it.

Exercise starts from day one. We don't want to build strength; we just want to keep the joint loose so that adhesions and stiffness do not result. The most likely bad result is inability to straighten the arm fully, so we want to pay particular attention to that motion. Exercise is passive and very simple. Straighten the arm out. Let it hang by your side. Flex it and let it straighten out again. Do this at least ten times at least twice a day, but don't force too hard at first. If the elbow is really tight, exercise in the shower with warm water running on the elbow. Then, twist the forearm. Start by extending your arm outward, palm facing the floor. Then turn your palm upward so that it

When to See the Doctor for Elbow Pain

- *Severe pain even when not moving arm.*
- *Associated fever.*
- *Associated significant injury.*
- *Rapid development of swelling without injury.*
- *Persistence after six weeks of home treatment.*

faces the ceiling. Repeat ten times, twice a day. As you get better, do the exercises faster and force them a little harder but don't force all the way. As soon as you feel the beginning of pain, back off.

If you are taking antiinflammatory drugs, remember to take them just as prescribed. If you have been lazy and skipped some doses, that might just be the cause of your flare-up.

WHAT TO EXPECT AT THE DOCTOR'S OFFICE

The elbow will be examined and taken through its range of motion. X-rays are likely if you have had an injury, but they are of little value otherwise. If the elbow is swollen, fluid may be withdrawn through a needle. This is quick, easy, and pretty safe and can give good information about gout or infection. You may be given a nonsteroidal, antiinflammatory drug or, if you are already taking one, the dosage may be increased. Injection with a corticosteroid can sometimes be helpful if the problem is one of inflammation, but injection has some hazard if the injection is around a tendon, because the tendon can be weakened by the medicine. At any rate, you shouldn't have more than an occasional injection. Surgery is rarely needed unless there is a fracture, in which case the bones may need to be surgically set and a pin may need to be placed. You may be sent to a physical therapist, but it is usually better for you to do your own exercises regularly rather than relying on professional treatment just a few times a week.

7/ *Pain in the Shoulder*

When the shoulder is affected by a problem, it has a tendency to become "frozen" regardless of the nature of the problem. The frozen shoulder is stiff, limited in motion, and can be permanently stiff if not appropriately treated. Understanding the way that the shoulder works will help you understand the many different injuries that result in the same general problem.

The shoulder is our largest non–weight-bearing joint. It has a complicated set of motions. Actually, the motions come from a series of three different joints that in combination give us the ability to swing our arms every which way together with reasonable strength and stability at the joint.

If you lift your arms straight up at the side over your head, you can feel the three joints come into play one after another by using your other hand to feel the movement of the bones. The first 90 degrees of motion, from arm at your side to arm straight out to the side, comes from the true shoulder joint. This joint is a shallow ball and socket held together by a tough fibrous capsule. It is covered over with tendons and muscles. It connects the arm to the shoulder blade. As you raise your arm higher, the shoulder blade itself begins to move, because of motion at a fibrous joint that joins the shoulder blade to the collar bone. This allows perhaps 75 degrees more of motion. Finally, the entire collar bone begins to tilt up, moving at a fibrous joint connecting the collar bone to the breast bone. This intricate design permits more motion at the shoulder joint than at any other joint.

An injury of any kind tends to immobilize this complex apparatus, and the inflammation that is helping repair the damage can involve nearby tissues. As healing occurs, scarring and adhesions may stick the surfaces together and motion can be permanently lost—hence the frozen shoulder.

This stiffening process is much more common in the shoulder than in any other joint. The causes can be many: injury, calcific tendonitis, rheumatoid arthritis, aseptic necrosis, ankylosing spondylitis, osteoarthritis, and many other conditions that start either in the joint itself or in the bursa or surrounding ligaments.

You won't have to see a doctor for most shoulder problems. However, be rather careful with the shoulder. If your home treatment is not progressing well, don't put off the doctor visit too long, or you may end up with a permanently stiff shoulder and a long series of treatments to loosen it up.

HOME TREATMENT

Treatment involves resting the sore area in combination with exercise to prevent adhesions and stiffness. It is the old problem of rest versus exercise, and you need both in carefully considered amounts. Rest means take it easy and listen to the pain message. Try not to do things that hurt or things that make the pain worse the next day. Avoid the activity that started the whole business. Common sense will help tell you what to do.

Better rest can be obtained with a sling (which is also

When to See the Doctor for Shoulder Pain

- *Severe pain when shoulder is at rest.*
- *Fever without flulike aches.*
- *Associated significant injury.*
- *Unable to lift the arms straight out to the side.*
- *Persistence after six weeks of home treatment.*

useful for elbow problems discussed in Problem 6). To fashion a sling, you need two big safety pins and a square piece of cloth two to three feet on a side. Fold the cloth diagonally to make a triangle. Put your forearm across the middle of the triangle with your wrist at the right-angle corner. Have a helper tie or pin the free ends of the triangle behind your neck. Pin up the triangular cravat around the elbow as if you were wrapping a package. This simple sling is the most important treatment for everything from a broken shoulder to acute calcific tendonitis. Wear it all the time for the first few days; then decrease use as the pain subsides.

Exercise is absolutely important, but it must be "passive." You are not trying to build strength, but rather to keep things loose. Work the shoulder through its normal motion in all directions, or as close to that goal as you can come without too much discomfort, several times each day. Stretch. Start with "pendulum swings," either dangling your bad arm off the bed or leaning over so that it can hang like a pendulum. Swing it around in little circles and let the circles enlarge. As you get better, you can do this exercise out to the side where it eventually becomes an "airplane propeller" movement. Try gentle hand claps, first in front of your chest, then over your head, then behind your back, then repeat. To note your progress, do "wall climbing." Here, you stand sideways to a wall at about a two-foot distance. With arms straight, walk your fingers up the wall. See how high you can get without too much pain. Make a mark, and try to beat it each day.

Aspirin, ibuprofen, or acetaminophen may be used to decrease pain, but stay free of major pain killers. If your doctor has prescribed antiinflammatory drugs, be sure that you are taking them exactly as prescribed.

WHAT TO EXPECT AT THE DOCTOR'S OFFICE

The doctor will examine the shoulder and its range of motion. X-rays may be taken and may show calcium deposits, but this is neither good nor bad, and having calcium deposits doesn't change the treatment. You may be given an antiinflammatory drug. You should be instructed in exercises, and you should set up a future appointment to make sure things are going well. If you don't do the exercises or if the doctor is not familiar with them, you may be sent to a physical therapist for instruction or treatment. The shoulder may be injected with a steroid—this often helps. In severe, late cases, the joint may be "mobilized under anesthesia" to loosen it up. This rather primitive approach can be surprisingly useful. Surgery is not helpful in most instances; for example, calcium removal is often unsuccessful and the problem recurs. The artificial shoulder joint is a promising approach for severe and persistent problems.

8/ *Pain in the Hip*

The hip is a "ball and socket" joint. The largest bone in the body, the femur, is in the thigh and narrows to a "neck" that angles into the pelvis and ends in a ball-shaped knob. This ball fits into a curved socket in the pelvic bones (acetabulum). This arrangement provides a joint that can move freely in all directions. The joint itself is located rather deeply under some big muscles so that it is protected from dislocating—that is, from coming out of the socket.

Two special problems arise because of this anatomical arrangement. The narrow neck of the femur can break rather easily, and this is usually what happens when an older person "breaks a hip" after a slight fall. Also, the "ball" part of the joint must get its blood supply from below, and the small artery that supplies the head of the femur can become clogged, leading to death of the bone and a kind of arthritis called aseptic necrosis.

The hip joint can also become infected. Very occasionally it will be the site for an attack of gout. The bursae that lie over the joint can be inflamed with bursitis. Rheumatoid arthritis can injure the joint. Conditions such as ankylosing spondylitis can cause stiffness or loss of motion of the hip.

A "flexion contracture" is a common consequence of hip problems. This means that motion of the hip joint has been partly lost. The hip becomes partially fixed in a slightly bent position. When walking or standing, this causes the pelvis to tilt forward, so that when you stand straight, the back has to curve a little more. This throws extra strain on the low back area.

For poorly understood reasons, pain in the hip is often felt down the leg, often at or just above the knee. This is called "referred" pain. Nonreferred hip pain may be felt in the groin or the upper outer thigh. Pain that starts in the lower back is often felt in the region of the hip. Since the hip joint is so deeply located, it can often be troublesome to locate the exact source of pain in these regions.

HOME TREATMENT

Listen for the pain message and try to avoid activities that are painful or that aggravate pain. You will want to avoid pain medication as much as possible. Rest the joint from painful activities. Use a cane or crutches if necessary. The cane is usually best held in the hand opposite to the painful hip, since this allows greater relaxation in the large muscles around the sore hip joint. Move the cane and the affected side simultaneously, then the good side, then repeat. As the pain begins to resolve, exercise should be gradually introduced. First use gentle motion exercises to free the hip and prevent stiffness. Stand with your good hip by a table and lean on the table with your hand. Let the bad hip swing to and fro and front and back. Lie on your back with your body half off the bed and the bad hip hanging and let the leg stretch backward toward the floor. See how far apart you can straddle your legs

When to See the Doctor for Hip Pain

- *Inability to walk.*
- *Associated fever.*
- *Severe pain when not bearing weight.*
- *Associated recent injury.*
- *Persistence after six weeks of home treatment.*

and bend the upper body from side to side. Try to turn your feet apart like a duck so that the rotation ligaments are stretched. Repeat these exercises gently two or three times a day.

Then introduce more active exercises to strengthen the muscles around the hips. Lie on your back and raise your legs. Swimming stretches muscles and builds good muscle tone. Bicycle or walk. When walking, start with short strides and gradually lengthen them as you loosen up. Gradually increase your effort and distance, but not by more than 10 percent each day. A good firm bed will help, and the best sleeping position is on your back. Avoid pillows beneath the knees or under the lower back. Make sure you are taking antiinflammatory medication as prescribed, especially if you have rheumatoid arthritis or ankylosing spondylitis.

WHAT TO EXPECT AT THE DOCTOR'S OFFICE

The hip will be examined and taken through its ranges of motion. Your other leg joints and back will also be examined. X-rays may well be necessary. Antiinflammatory medication may be prescribed or the dosage increased. Injection is only rarely used or needed. One of several surgical procedures may be recommended if the pain is bad and persistent or if you are having real problems walking, and time and home treatment have not solved the problem. Total hip replacement is a remarkable operation and has largely superceded many older techniques. This operation is almost always successful in stopping pain and may help mobility a great deal. The artificial hip should last at least 10 to 15 years with current techniques. You get up and around quite quickly after surgery, and complications are relatively rare. Most golfers are able to get back on the golf course. Other older procedures include pinning of the hip, replacing either the ball or the socket, but not both, or removing a wedge of bone to straighten out the joint angle.

9/ *Pain in the Knee*

The knee is a hinge. It is a large weight-bearing joint, but its motion is much more strictly limited than that of most other joints. It will straighten to make the leg a stable support, and it will bend to more than a right angle, to approximately 120 degrees. However, it will not move in any other direction. The limited motion of the knee gives it great strength, but it is not engineered to take side stresses.

There are two cartilage compartments in the knee, one inner and one outer. If the cartilage wears unevenly, the leg can bow in or bow out, or if you were born with crooked legs, there can be strain that causes the cartilage to wear more rapidly. If you are overweight, you are far more likely to have knee problems.

The knee must be stable, and it must be able to extend fully to a straight leg. If it lacks full extension, the muscles have to support the body at all times and strain is continuous. Normally, our knee locks in the straight position and allows us to rest. Horses are able to sleep standing up because they can rest on their knees. If the knee wobbles from side to side, there is too much stress on the side ligaments, and the condition may gradually worsen.

If the knee is unstable and wobbles or if it cannot be straightened out, you need the doctor. Similarly, you need a physician if there is a possibility of gout or an infection; the knee is the joint most frequently bothered by these serious problems. Finally, if there is pain or swelling in the calf below the sore knee, you may have a blood clot, but more likely you have a "Baker cyst," and you need the doctor. These cysts start as fluid-filled sacs in an inflamed knee but enlarge through the tissues of the calf and may cause swelling quite a distance below the knee.

Many people have wondered if exercise such as walking or running can cause knee problems. No. If the knee is not injured, exercise and weight-bearing is good for the knee. It helps nourish the cartilage, and it keeps the side ligaments, the muscles, and the bones strong—this helps keep the knee stable.

HOME TREATMENT

Listen to the pain message and try not to do things that aggravate the pain either immediately or the next day. If there has been a recent injury, then an elastic bandage may help; otherwise, probably not. Using a cane can help; the cane is best carried in the hand on the side of the painful knee by most, while some carry it on the opposite side.

Do not use a pillow under the knee at night or at any other time, as this can make the knee stiffen so that it cannot be straightened out.

Exercises should be started slowly and performed several times daily if possible. Swimming is good, because there is no weight-bearing requirement. From the beginning pay close attention to flexing and straightening the leg. A friend can help, since it may be more comfortable to move the leg passively. But work at getting

When to See the Doctor for Knee Pain

- *Unable to walk at all.*
- *Rapid development of swelling without injury.*
- *Associated fever.*
- *Associated recent injury and the knee wobbles from side to side or can't be straightened.*
- *Severe pain when not bearing weight.*
- *Pain and swelling in the calf below a swollen or painful knee.*
- *Persistence after six weeks of home treatment.*

it straight and keeping it straight. Next begin isometric exercises. Tense the muscles in your upper leg, front and back, at the same time, so that you are exerting force but your leg is not moving. Exert the force for two seconds, then rest two seconds. Do ten repetitions three times a day. Then begin gentle active exercises. A bicycle in a low gear is a good place to start. Stationary bicycles are fine. Be sure that the seat is relatively high; your knee should not bend to more than a right angle during the bicycle stroke. Walking is probably the best overall exercise, and distances should be gradually increased. Avoid exercises or activities that simulate deep knee bends, as they place too much stress on the knee. Knee problems can come from the feet. Proper shoes, as discussed in the next three sections, can help.

Make sure that you are taking any prescribed medication as directed, since your painful knee could be caused by too little medication.

WHAT TO EXPECT AT THE DOCTOR'S OFFICE

The knee and other joints will be examined and taken through their range of motion. An x-ray of the knee may be taken. If a Baker cyst is suspected, or for diagnostic reasons, some fluid may be drawn from the knee through a needle and tested. This procedure is easy, not too uncomfortable, and quite safe. There are a number of operations that are quite helpful for knee problems. A torn meniscus may be removed, or the cartilage may be shaved through arthroscopic surgery. Increasingly, doctors are using the arthroscope to visualize knee problems and often to help it. This is a minor and easy procedure. For severe and persistent problems, total knee replacement may be recommended. This is an excellent operation and usually gives total pain relief. Next to the hip, knee replacement is the most successful total joint replacement surgery.

10/ *Pain in the Ankle*

The ankle is a large weight-bearing joint that is unavoidably stressed at each step. It can be involved by several kinds of arthritis, but pain and instability are more frequently a result of problems in the ligaments near the joints. The sprained ankle is a simple example of this. With an ankle sprain, the ligament attaching the bump on the outer side of the ankle to the outer surface of the foot is injured at one or both ends. The ankle itself is all right. With arthritis, the ligaments may have been injured so that the joint slips and wobbles. This results in further stress on the ligaments, and pain and instability result. Walking on an unstable joint just increases the damage, but if you can stabilize the joint, walking is usually all right.

If you look down your leg when you are lying and again when you are standing, you can tell if the joint is stable. If it is unstable, the line of weight going down your leg will not be straight down the foot when you stand. Perhaps the foot will be slipped to a half inch or an inch to the outside or inside of where it should be. When you are not bearing weight, it will move back in line toward a more normal position. The unstable joint may actually slip sideways if you try to move the foot with your hands.

HOME TREATMENT

Listen to the pain message; it is telling you to rest the part a bit more, to provide support for the unstable ankle, to back off on your exercise progression, or to use an aid to take weight off the ankle. The unstable ankle should be supported for major weight-bearing activity. Instability does not mean just a swollen ankle; it means the ankle is displaced sideways or is crooked. Support is most simply obtained by high-lacing boots, but sometimes these will be too uncomfortable and you will have to have specially made boots or an ankle brace. Professional help is required for adequate fitting of such devices, and they can be quite expensive.

For the stable ankle, an elastic bandage and a shoe with a comfortable, thick heel pad will help. Jogging shoes (described in problems 11 and 12) are good. Recently, very light hiking boots that are just like running shoes but go above the ankle have become available, and these are often excellent; they give more support.

Crutches are often a big help for a flare-up, and even a cane can help you take the weight off the sore ankle. Remember to have the crutches short enough so as not to injure the nerves in your armpits by leaning on the crutch; take the weight on your hands or arms.

If you have a true arthritis, make particularly sure that you have been taking any prescribed medication exactly. Sometimes a patient gets a little bored and lax with the pill-taking routine and a few days later experiences difficulty walking because of pain or swelling.

As soon as the pain begins to decrease, you can gently begin to exercise the joint again. Swimming is good, because you don't have to bear weight. Start easily

When to See the Doctor for Ankle Pain

- *Unable to walk.*
- *Associated fever.*
- *Severe pain when not bearing weight.*
- *Heat and redness in the area of pain.*
- *Persistence after six weeks of home treatment.*

and slowly with your exercises. Sit on a chair, let the leg hang free, and wiggle the foot up and down and in and out. Later, walk carefully with an ankle bandage for support. Stretch the ankle by putting the forefoot on a step and lowering the heel. As the ankle gains strength, you can walk on tip toe and walk on your heels to stretch and strengthen the joint. Do the exercises several times a day; the ankle shouldn't be a lot worse after the exercise if you aren't overdoing it. Keep at it, but take your time and be patient as well.

WHAT TO EXPECT AT THE DOCTOR'S OFFICE

The ankle and the area around it will be examined. X-rays may be necessary. Antiinflammatory medications may be prescribed or the dosage increased. Special shoes or braces may be prescribed. Surgery is occasionally necessary. Fusion of the ankle is the most generally useful procedure; a fixed, pain-free ankle is far preferable to an unstable and painful one. The artificial ankle joint is not yet satisfactory for most people, but progress is rapid in this area.

11/ *Pain in the Heel*

Heel pain can occur at one of two places; the bottom of the heel or the back of the heel. The heel bone, the calcaneus, is the largest bone of the foot and bears our full weight during part of each stride. The painful heel, in almost all instances, is caused by excessive strain on one of the two major ligaments, and the pain occurs where these ligaments attach. The Achilles tendon attaches at the back of the heel. This is the strongest tendon in the body and connects the muscles on the back of the calf to the heel. The force of contraction of the muscles enables us to stand on tiptoe and gives an extra thrust as we walk. Damage to this tendon attachment is called Achilles tendonitis. Frequently, there will also be tears in the tendon itself or in the lower part of the muscle.

The heel spur syndrome affects the bottom of the heel. This is where the ligaments that make up the arch of the foot attach to the heel bone. These ligaments function like a bowstring to arch the foot, so they are under pressure every time we stand or step. If the problem persists, calcium may develop in the inflamed area where the ligaments attach. The presence of the calcium spur may or may not cause additional pain; often the calcium spur itself is only part of a painful process. Many people have pain without visible spurs on x-ray, while others have spurs but no pain.

Usually heel pain is a simple result of a minor and forgotten injury. Unfortunately, since we strain the injured part every time we walk or stand, these problems can become a vicious cycle in which there is more injury, more inflammation, more injury, and so forth.

HOME TREATMENT

Rest, avoidance of further injury, and gradual resumption of activity as the pain subsides are indicated. Activities not requiring weight bearing, like swimming, can be continued full tilt.

For Achilles tendonitis, rest the foot or feet. Use a shoe with a high heel wedge and a lot of padding, since this limits the stretch on the tendon. Warm up and stretch carefully for 10 to 15 minutes before activities that might cause reinjury. Exercises such as tennis or walking uphill are not good; these stress the tendon. Remember that tight muscles on the back of the leg put extra strain on this tendon, so warm up with toe-touching or other stretching exercises for the calf muscles.

For the heel spur syndrome, treatment is just the same, except that the activities to avoid are ones that cause pounding on the bottom of the heel. Heel padding will help, but support for the arch is even more important, since this takes tension off the ligaments whose job it is to hold the arch. Commercially made running shoes are often very helpful. In most of these shoes, the cushioning air cells break down after a few months, so you should change shoes even before they appear worn out. The new shoes that have a big air cushion under the arch and the heel are excellent and will last

When to See the Doctor for Heel Pain

- *Unable to walk.*
- *Associated fever.*
- *Areas of numbness or tingling.*
- *Heat or redness in the area of pain.*
- *Severe pain when not bearing weight.*
- *Persistence after six weeks of home treatment.*

longer without losing their energy-absorbing properties. Don't worry about wearing a "silly-looking" shoe; forget fashion and concentrate on getting well. This kind of problem can take a year or more to resolve, or it may go away quickly. Keep trying.

WHAT TO EXPECT AT THE DOCTOR'S OFFICE

Your doctor will examine the painful areas and give you advice on home treatment. If a significant form of arthritis such as Reiter's syndrome or ankylosing spondylitis, which can result in heel pain, is present, major relief may be obtained from indomethacin or other nonsteroidal, antiinflammatory agents. These drugs should not be used for injuries as a rule, since they suppress the healing inflammatory response. Injection of steroids into the Achilles tendon area is quite dangerous and should be avoided; the entire tendon will sometimes rip apart after an injection has weakened it. Some doctors have found it helpful to scrape the heel spur off the underlying bone with a needle or a knife; this procedure has also met with mixed success. X-rays or bone scans may be taken but are not usually necessary.

12/ *Pain in the Ball of the Foot*

The sole of your shoe wears most rapidly at the ball of your foot, and your shoe may get a hole in it at that point. This is the point of greatest stress when we walk. We make it even worse by wearing footwear designed for fashion rather than function. And, unfortunately, this area is where the metatarsal bones join the toe bones; there are five important joints in this region in each foot. At these "MTP" or metatarsal-phalangeal joints a great proportion of the arthritis that affects the foot occurs.

The consequences of arthritis in the forefoot (metatarsalgia) are major and adverse. With every step we place weight on this area, and it is difficult indeed to walk without using the forefoot. Even a small problem can make walking difficult, and then the other muscles, tendons, ligaments, and bones begin to lose strength. Serious attention is required because your careful work at home can pay major dividends. Even people with major kinds of arthritis will find that attention to local factors here can make all the difference.

HOME TREATMENT

The basic principle is quite simple. The idea is to move the weight-bearing burden away from the painful part so that the inflammation can subside and the part can heal. The metatarsal bar, a strip of sole leather that the shoemaker sews or glues on about an inch behind the contact point where you are wearing out the sole, is an important device to shift your weight. An insert in the shoe to do the same thing takes up room in the shoe, and most feet with arthritis need more room rather than less; but inserts help some people and have the advantage that they can be transferred from shoe to shoe. The metatarsal bar goes on the outside of the shoe. When you check your area of greatest pain against the area of greatest wear on the shoe, you will find that they are at the same place. Press on your foot about an inch behind the sore place, and you will note how much better it feels and how the toes line up straighter. The metatarsal bar will also help your arch. It is an inexpensive device, and any good shoemaker knows how to fit one. Fix several pairs of shoes.

Good shoes are critical to problems of foot pain. Don't wear shoes with pointed toes. Women should avoid high heels—they throw additional weight on the forefoot. Look for a wide toe box in a shoe. You can tell a lot in the store by walking around before buying; don't go home with a purchase that isn't comfortable no matter what the salesperson says. Ask particularly to try the "Duckbill" made by the Joyce Company or the "Roundabout" by Dr. Scholl. These shoes have a wide toe box and are comfortable for most; they are readily available, and their cost is much less than that of specially made shoes. Try the athletic shoe department for casual shoes. The newer shoes designed for long-distance running on pavement are excellent for arthritis and should be more widely used; they are comfortable and relatively inexpensive. Look for shoes

When to See the Doctor for Pain in the Ball of the Foot

- *Unable to walk at all.*
- *Associated fever.*
- *Heat or redness at the area of pain.*
- *Areas of numbness or tingling.*
- *Significant injury.*
- *Severe pain when not bearing weight.*
- *Persistence after six weeks of home treatment.*

with a good heel wedge support, a nylon upper that will spread in the toe box, and laces that run through guides rather than eyelets so that they adjust smoothly. The new shoes with air cushions seem particular satisfactory for many people.

If your problem with pain in the forefoot occurs at night, you will need something to raise the covers off the foot. A pillow under the covers at the bottom of the bed is the easiest solution; a side-lying *L*-shaped piece of wood may be better for tall people.

WHAT TO EXPECT AT THE DOCTOR'S OFFICE

The doctor will examine your foot and ankle and sometimes take an x-ray. The advice will be much the same as that given above. Injection of the area is only occasionally of some use. Fancy shoes may be ordered, but if you have followed the instructions under "Home Treatment," you are likely to be disappointed when the $400 shoes are not as comfortable as those selected in a shoe store.

If problems are persistent, surgery is sometimes required and is often very worthwhile. Bunionectomy, metatarsal head resection, and resection of a Morton's neuroma (nerve tumor) are three frequently useful procedures. The operation for putting plastic joints in the forefoot is not yet perfected. Finally, your doctor may recommend antiinflammatory medications to improve an underlying arthritis.

13/ *Pain at Night*

Night pain is usually an indication of the severity of pain. Usually pain will decrease at night as the body diminishes its sensation input for sleep and the body becomes less active. Typically a patient with arthritis may have occasional night pain when changing position but will be free of serious discomfort for most of the night. While it may seem that sleep is lost during these brief episodes, the body actually gets plenty of rest and no serious problem is present.

Most people overestimate the magnitude of a sleeping problem. Indeed, we have been characterized as a nation of insomniacs. The worry makes it worse. Unless the sleeping time totals less than four hours, the body is very good at substituting quality for quantity. The drive to sleep is overwhelming, and the truly tired person will sleep even under adverse circumstances. Once in a great while, a vicious cycle occurs in which pain prevents sleep, fatigue prevents rational approaches to problems during the day, depression aggravates pain, and sleep is even more disturbed by pain and depression the following night. The hints given here are reasonably obvious, but they can help with most of these problems.

HOME TREATMENT

Consult the previous sections for techniques for dealing with pain in specific body locations.

Have a comfortable bed. Usually a moderately firm mattress of good quality is the best choice. A water bed, which supports the weight of the body evenly and can be kept quite warm, is successful for some people. Others can never get used to the thing. Pillows can be used here and there to increase comfort. For example, they can be placed on the sides to limit turning, under the neck, under the lower back, or below the feet to keep covers off the feet. Be careful not to use a pillow under the knees if there is any problem with the knee or hips, as stiffness and contracture can result.

Don't go to bed early to try to ensure enough sleep. Wait until you're tired. You want your body so ready for sleep that it suppresses painful signals from the nerves.

Beware of sedatives and sleeping pills. These give the wrong kind of sleep, cause rebound depression, tend to be habit-forming, and only very rarely help solve sleeping problems.

Beware also of pain-killing drugs. These do not affect the arthritis or pain but only suppress the symptoms, and the symptom of night pain is one that should be listened to. The body has mechanisms for adjusting to long-term pain, and many doctors feel that pain medications actually interfere with normal adaptation to pain.

The sleeping partner is important. A restless partner may make twin beds advisable. On the other hand, sexual relations at bedtime encourage good relaxation and healthy sleep.

A glass of warm nonfat milk at bedtime helps many people. Generally it is good not to have eaten for two or more hours before retiring.

When to See the Doctor for Pain at Night

- *Pain does not allow a total of four hours of sleep at night.*
- *Pain persists after six weeks of home treatment.*

Red wine or whiskey in the late evening are particular enemies of sleep. The ingredients in many common cold remedies can make it difficult for some people to sleep. And be careful, of course, to avoid caffeinated coffee. Be sure to take any antiinflammatory drugs as prescribed. If your doctor has encouraged you to adjust your own doses, try to increase the number of times each day that you take the medication, and be sure that you have a dose at bedtime. Setting the alarm so you can take another dose in the middle of the night may be worthwhile.

Leg cramps are another common problem. Be sure that you are taking your calcium supplements. Try a warm bath before bedtime. Walk and exercise moderately during the day and do stretching exercises to stretch out the muscles before going to bed. Avoid active exercises within two hours of bedtime.

WHAT TO EXPECT AT THE DOCTOR'S OFFICE

The complaint of night pain is a signal to your doctor that your pain syndrome may need some extra attention. Examination, tests, even x-rays may be required. A new treatment program may be developed, emphasizing more powerful anti-inflammatory medicines. Quinine or Benadryl may be helpful for problems of leg cramps or the "restless leg" syndrome in which pain or a crawling sensation on the skin makes you get up and walk around in the middle of the night for relief.

14/ *Pain after Exercise*

We all get stiff after unusual exertion, and as we grow older we get stiffer more easily. Often the stiffness will be maximum on the second to fifth day after the exercise. This results in a paradox. In order to stay in good physical shape, we all will have substantial amounts of pain and stiffness from time to time. To relieve this kind of discomfort, you have to increase your exercise, and this inevitably triggers at least a few episodes of increased pain. This is not a message to eliminate the exercise program. Rather, it is a suggestion from your body to proceed more carefully with a gentle exercise progression. So don't be discouraged by pain after exercise. Listen to the pain message and work with it.

On the other hand, people with osteoarthritis have pain during exercise that usually is relieved by rest. If you have significant arthritis, the pain after exercise may be localized to the joints and not the muscles; if the pain lasts more than two hours after you have stopped exercising, you may need to rethink your exercise program. You don't need the doctor unless signs of severe injury or nerve damage are present or unless the problem continues to bother you quite a bit for quite a while. This problem is a signal to review your home exercise program.

HOME TREATMENT

Almost always, pain after exercise indicates that you have disregarded one of the principles of a sound exercise program. Let's review them.

Exercise should not make you hurt very much. Don't try to exercise through pain. If you hurt after exercise, that exercise is a bit too much for you right now.

Exercise programs should be daily. The weekend gardener is not going to become fit or able, may have reinjury, and will experience increased pain and stiffness on following days.

Exercise programs should be gently graded. No day's activities should be more than a 10 percent increase over the typical day's activity. Slow and steady progression is essential to success. Exercise programs should emphasize smooth actions, as with swimming, walking, or bicycling, until good conditioning is achieved. Jerky exercises with incompletely trained muscles are likely to result in reinjury.

Exercise programs should emphasize suppleness and muscle tone, not absolute strength. The stress of lifting heavy objects, squeezing balls, and so forth is likely to damage an already injured joint. Swimming easily is an excellent exercise. Exercise should be preceded by a warm-up period in which the joints, ligaments, and muscles are stretched gently. The parts to be used should be physically warm; on a cold day, wear warm clothing.

Exercise programs are in addition to, not instead of, prescribed medications.

Exercise programs always have setbacks in which there

When to See the Doctor for Pain after Exercise

- *Inability to move the part at all.*
- *Numbness or tingling in an arm or a leg.*
- *Persistence of this pain pattern for more than three months.*

are periods of increased pain. This does not mean that the idea is wrong. Back off just a little bit and begin again more gently.

WHAT TO EXPECT AT THE DOCTOR'S OFFICE

The physician will reinforce the basic exercise concepts. If you have trouble figuring out how to apply the principles in your own life, you may be referred to a physical therapist. Antiinflammatory medication may be prescribed or the dosage may be increased. If your physician does not try to help you find ways to exercise safely and comfortably, try to find another physician who can help you. Older people are likely to think that serious exercise programs are for the young. This is absolutely not so—the principles of conditioning apply to all ages. You won't get as well as you might unless you persevere in your exercise program.

15/ *Problems with Fatigue*

Most older people experience, at some time, some degree of fatigue. But most problems with fatigue are not physical weakness; they are related to failure to exercise, depression, unhappiness, worry, or boredom. True weakness, as with inability to move an arm or a leg, is a physical problem involving nerves, brain, or muscle and needs immediate medical attention. Fatigue or tiredness is far more common than true weakness.

Another common cause for fatigue is overuse of one drug or another. For example, excess caffeine intake leading to poor sleep habits can cause daytime fatigue. Or tranquilizers can make you feel tired or drowsy. Once the normal sleep cycle has been disturbed, there is a tendency to grab an afternoon nap. Then the following night's sleep is not good, because the afternoon nap decreased the need for sleep at night. A vicious cycle has been set in motion.

You may be assuming from this discussion that most fatigue is not serious. Usually that is correct. Even when arthritis is associated, most fatigue results from misunderstanding your body. Reestablishing a pattern of healthy activity, more moderate drug use, and good nocturnal sleep will do wonders.

But if you have an inflammatory arthritis, such as rheumatoid arthritis or lupus, the disease may be causing the fatigue. This is a more serious kind of fatigue, and improving your living patterns will not help much. In such cases the "sed rate" is elevated and there may be a low-grade fever. A hematocrit test may show the anemia of chronic disease. There may be some weight loss. Treatment of this kind of disease is based on treating the disease causing the fatigue; it may take some time to treat it correctly.

When you mention fatigue, most people don't even think of the problems just described. Instead they think of a problem with the thyroid, hypoglycemia, or anemia. These are so unusual as causes of fatigue that you can almost forget about them. But if your fatigue persists more than six weeks despite home treatment, your doctor might want to check out these and other possibilities or may be able to reassure you that these problems are not present.

Fatigue is not a symptom of old age. In fact, as you get older, you need less sleep and tend to be more alert, particularly early in the day. So pay attention to this symptom.

HOME TREATMENT

Listen to the fatigue message from your body. Heed it, but don't give in to it. Rest if you are tired, but alternate such periods with times of activity. Fatigue, because it can lead to physical deconditioning, can become its own cause.

Decrease all possible drugs including caffeine, nicotine, alcohol, tranquilizers, and probably television. Ingredients in common cold or allergy medications can cause fatigue, as can Valium and codeine. Suspect all drugs.

Increase new activities. Friends, hobbies, travel,

When to See the Doctor for Problems of Fatigue

- *Associated weight loss or fever.*
- *Weakness—not tiredness.*
- *Fatigue preventing you from doing your usual activities.*
- *Fatigue and tiredness lasting more than six weeks.*

vacations, and even shopping tend to break the fatigue cycle. Increase your activity level by addition of smooth, graded, and easy exercises. Exercise helps you become involved in new and different things as well as giving physical help by increasing your stamina.

Expect improvement to be slow and to be discouraged at times. Persevere.

WHAT TO EXPECT AT THE DOCTOR'S OFFICE

The topics previously noted should be explored in depth at the doctor's office with particular attention to the drugs being taken and to associated psychological events. The nerves and muscles will be the focus of the physical examination. Blood tests, including thyroid tests, hematocrit, sedimentation rate, and others may be ordered. Probably no abnormality will be found. If your doctor doesn't think the tests are necessary, don't insist.

Treatment will be essentially as described above. The doctor will treat the fatigue by treating the disease underlying. Do not expect to be given pep pills, tonics, vitamins, or other magic, and be patient.

16/ *Stiffness in the Morning*

Morning stiffness in the muscles and joints is the hallmark of inflammatory kinds of arthritis. With a sprained ankle, with rheumatoid arthritis, with ankylosing spondylitis, or with other kinds of inflammation, you may notice that the sore area is stiff in the morning but loosens up as the day goes on. This phenomenon is most pronounced in rheumatoid arthritis, in which morning stiffness generally lasts for an hour or more and can be a great aggravation. With osteoarthritis the stiffness usually lasts only a few moments.

No one really understands the reason for morning stiffness. Presumably, while the body is inactive, fluid leaks out from the small blood vessels and capillaries and the tissues become waterlogged. Then, if you try to move the part, the swollen tissues feel stiff until the motion pumps the fluid out through the lymph channels and the veins. If you sit or lie down during the day, the stiffness may return. This phenomenon is called "gelling" or the "gel phenomenon" after the behavior of gelatin, which remains liquid if kept moving and warm but solidifies if it sits for long. The phenomenon appears to be normal, but in the patient with inflammatory arthritis, it can be very vexing.

Don't let morning stiffness keep you in bed. If your stiffness is that severe, call the doctor and discuss the problem today.

HOME TREATMENT

With a minor local condition, such as a sprained ankle or a tennis elbow, don't worry about the stiffness. Think of it as a normal part of the process of bringing healing materials to the injured area. Loosen up carefully before activities and keep in mind that the healing is not yet complete. You should continue to protect the injured part.

With a condition like rheumatoid arthritis, the stiffness is apt to persist and you are going to have to come to grips with the problem. Use all the tricks you can to reduce the inflammation and the stiffness.

Be sure that you take any prescribed medication strictly according to schedule. Morning stiffness can be a sign of the activity of an arthritis, and the best way to reduce stiffness is to treat the arthritis. Your stiffness may be a signal that you have been sloppy in taking prescribed drugs. Or you may need more medication or a different drug. In particular, don't forget to take the last dose in the evening.

Ask your doctor about changing your medication schedule. Perhaps you can take a drug later in the evening or in the middle of the night so that there is medication in your blood in the morning when you are most stiff. If you are taking aspirin, some patients find that taking a coated aspirin (ecotrin, Enseals) immediately before retiring helps reduce the morning stiffness. These coated aspirin are absorbed more slowly, and the aspirin level lasts a bit longer. Avoid pain killers—they don't help morning stiffness. Stretch

When to See the Doctor for Morning Stiffness

- *The stiffness keeps you from getting out of bed at all.*
- *The problem persists longer than six weeks.*

gloves, of Spandex or similar elastic material, may help morning stiffness in the hands if worn overnight. Give them a try; the idea is to prevent the tissues from becoming waterlogged. Try a warm bath or shower upon arising. Work at gentle exercises in the bed before you get up. You will have a certain amount of stiffness each day, and you might as well get it worked out as soon as possible. Some people find that they are helped by using an electric blanket.

WHAT TO EXPECT AT THE DOCTOR'S OFFICE

The doctor's attention will be directed at control of the inflammation that is causing the stiffness. There may well be an increase in your prescribed medication or a change to a different set of treatments. For example, patients with rheumatoid arthritis may have their morning stiffness greatly helped by gold injections, penicillamine, or methotrexate.

Formal physical therapy programs are not likely to help, since this stiffness usually will have worked out by the time you reach the therapist. With an inflammatory arthritis condition, increased morning stiffness is a signal for increased attention on the part of both you and the doctor.

17/ *Spots, Wrinkles, and Baldness*

Our aging skins present a lot of superficial problems. The problems result from a combination of two factors. First, as we age we lose elasticity in the skin. The skin develops a greater portion of scar tissue and it does not spring back as quickly into a smooth contour. Second, damage from the sun accumulates over our lifetime and causes additional problems in the sun-exposed areas of our body. The aging skin lets air leak into the hair follicles so that the hair turns white. Some or all hair follicles lose the ability to produce hairs at all and the hair thins or balds. The loss of elasticity means that things tend to sag and crinkles in the face turn into deeper fixed wrinkles.

In general, you need not worry about these problems. The aging face can be considered as showing character as well as developing wrinkles. Thinning hair and baldness are not diseases, nor are aging spots.

Aging spots are pigmentary changes in the skin without medical significance. Some cells lose the ability to produce the pigment melanin, while others produce a bit too much of it. These changes can be thought of as an adult form of freckles. The most important medical observation is whether the skin in the area of a spot is thickened or not. If you run your fingers over the spot of concern with your eyes closed, can you feel it and tell where it is? If you can, then go to the discussion of the following problem, "Lumps and Bumps."

HOME TREATMENT

Stay out of the sun and use a sunscreen. This is particularly important if you are fair-skinned since such skin is far more prone to sun damage. Outside of this, there is not really very much you can do at home for these problems except not to worry about them.

WHAT TO EXPECT AT THE DOCTOR'S OFFICE

There are good medical approaches to the "problems" of aging skin, but they are entirely optional. Many people prefer their natural aging appearance to artificial cosmetic device. Others, who can afford it, elect to fight the aging stereotype by a variety of measures designed to preserve a more youthful appearance. Alternatives currently available are quite safe but also quite expensive. The choices range all the way from hair rinses to "keep the grey out" to an elaborate series of elective plastic surgical operations.

Perhaps you want to go the expensive route. You will probably want to see a dermatologist first, and then perhaps, a plastic surgeon. The dermatologist is likely to be more familiar with the effective cosmetic interventions than is a family physician or internist. (The dermatologist is also the key person to take care of any lumps and bumps that you are concerned about.) The most effective approaches to these problems, among a huge variety of not-so-good treatments, are Retin-A for

When to See the Doctor for Minor Skin Problems

- *Problem is a lump or a bump. (See Problem 18 first.)*
- *Consultation about wrinkle creams.*
- *Consultation about possible plastic surgery.*
- *Consultation about hair tonics or transplants.*

wrinkles and minoxodil for hair growth. Retin-A is the first wrinkle cream that actually works, and minoxodil does cause new hair to grow over previously bald spots. Unfortunately, Retin-A doesn't seem to work very well with old, fixed wrinkles, it sensitizes to the sun, and it dries the skin out. The new minoxodil hair isn't usually everything that you would want, it is unusual to grow back very much hair, and the older you are the less well it works.

The plastic surgeon can take out wrinkles by removing skin and stretching the remaining skin tighter. Many procedures are available. Wrinkles around the eyes can be taken out, as can bags under the eyes. A full "face lift" tightens the skin over the entire face. Sagging breasts can be reduced in size and lifted. Tucks can be taken in the tummy. Liposuction can remove fat, although the result usually is a little lumpy. Hair transplants can be partially effective in some people. Again, in good hands, done by a surgeon who performs the procedure often, these operations are quite safe. However, they are expensive, there is pain and discomfort involved, there is an occasional serious operative or perioperative mishap, and with some of the procedures you can't be seen in public for a week or so after the operation.

18/ *Lumps and Bumps*

The first test to apply to see if a skin problem warrants concern at all is whether the problem is a lump or a bump. If the skin is not thickened so that you can feel it with your eyes closed, it is very unlikely to be anything serious. The serious worry, of course, is cancer. Cancer is a terrifying word, and even though skin cancers are not very often serious, you still want to be alert to their occurrence.

The vast majority of lumps and bumps that develop with age are not skin cancers. They can be so-called senile keratoses, greyish, raised, flat, scaly lesions, or they can be warts, or skin tags (little, wobbly tags of skin that are actually benign papillomas).

There are three types of skin cancers, and all of them are quite common. Each year in the United States there are 25,000 cases of malignant melanoma, 100,000 of squamous cell carcinoma of the skin, and 400,000 of basal cell carcinomas of the skin. These are the most common cancers that occur, and one out of seven individuals will have a skin cancer at some point during his or her life. Fortunately, most of these are not very serious. With the exception of melanoma, they very seldom have metastases and hence can be completely cured in almost all cases by simple office procedures.

Malignant melanoma is potentially the most serious skin cancer, and as many as 5,800 deaths per year due to this cause are recorded in the United States each year. We tend to think of these cancers as moles that have turned black due to the fact that the tumor cells secrete melanin, the dark skin pigment. Dermatologists talk about the *A, B, C, D*'s of diagnoses of malignant melanoma, however. *A* stands for asymmetry, in which the lesion is not round but lopsided in appearance. *B* is for the border irregularity, much like the coast line of a country. *C* is for color irregularity, with some sections dark or black and others somewhat lighter. *D* is for the diameter, which is almost always over 6 mm, larger than the size of the eraser of a pencil. If you have a skin blemish that you think might be a melanoma, you should make an appointment to see a dermatologist for confirmation and treatment. You should not delay on this one.

Basal cell carcinomas almost never metastasize. When they get large, they are called "rodent ulcers" since they look like a little hole that something has been gnawing at. Earlier, they are translucent, with an appearance that has been likened to that of apple jelly. Early on these are quite innocent-looking lesions, but they don't go away and they are quite likely to bleed now and then over time.

Squamous cell carcinomas come from malignant change in the most superficial cells of the skin and can take a number of appearances. However, they persist and grow slowly in size. Frequently, they will ulcerate and bleed. These can also occur inside the mouth and on the tongue, particularly in smokers.

When to See the Doctor for Skin Lumps or Bumps

- *A skin blemish that you think might be a malignant melanoma.*
- *Any sore that won't heal.*
- *Any mouth lesions that won't heal, particularly if you have been a smoker.*

HOME TREATMENT

Prevention is always the best policy. All these skin cancers are more common in fair-skinned individuals and all are associated with sun exposure. Use a floppy, broad-brimmed hat, avoid strong and long sun exposure, and use sunscreens when you are out in the sun. You will slow down the aging of the skin and improve cosmetic appearance as well.

You need to regularly examine your body, perhaps every several months, to see if any new changes have occurred in your skin. Be aware of your body, and you will detect lesions early enough so that they won't be a problem. For smokers, if you have stopped smoking for a few years, your risk of mouth and tongue cancer goes back nearly to normal. But anyone who ever has smoked cigarettes, pipes, or cigars should examine the inside of the mouth and the tongue with a flashlight at least every few months. Be alert, again, for development of changes, either white plaques or sores that won't heal. Squamous cell cancers of the lips or mouth are more serious than those of the skin, and you want to be absolutely sure that any suspicious lesion is checked out right away.

WHAT TO EXPECT AT THE DOCTOR'S OFFICE

You are going to need a dermatologist for these problems in most areas of the country. The dermatologist is considerably more adept at making the diagnosis than most general physicians and can biopsy and often cure the problem all at the same visit. Some of these cancers can be cured entirely with an electric current and don't even require surgery. One thing to remember: If you get one of these cancers, you are quite likely to get another. So, once you have had the first one cured, it is a good idea to have regular examinations to make sure that nothing new has developed. Subsequent problems are not recurrences of the same cancer; they usually are brand new cancers arising because of the same causes—aging skin and sun exposure.

19/ *Chest Pain*

Chest pain is a serious symptom meaning "heart attack" to most people. Serious chest discomfort should usually be evaluated by a physician.

While pain from the heart may sometimes be mild, it is usually intense. Sometimes a feeling of pressure or squeezing on the chest is more prominent than actual pain. Almost always, the pain or discomfort will be felt in part below the breast bone. It may also be felt in the jaw or down the inner part of either arm. There may be nausea and sweating. If dizziness, shortness of breath or irregularity of the pulse is present, it is particularly important that a physician be seen *immediately*.

A related form of heart pain is not a heart attack but is termed "angina pectoris" or "angina." These pains also can occur in the upper arms or the jaw, but usually involve part of the breast bone (sternum). Angina pains occur with exercise and sometimes with stress, and they go away with rest and relaxation. They are a result of narrowed arteries to the heart that are unable to supply enough blood when the heart is working hard. In a heart attack, one of these same arteries has actually become totally blocked.

However, all chest pain does not come from the heart. Pain can also come from the chest wall (including muscles, ligaments, ribs, and rib cartilage), the lungs, the outside covering of the lungs (pleurisy), the outside covering of the heart (pericarditis), the esophagus, the diaphragm, the spine, the skin, or the organs in the upper part of the abdomen. Often it is difficult even for a physician to determine the precise origin of the pain. Therefore there are no absolute rules that enable you to determine which pains may be treated at home. The following guidelines usually work and are used by doctors, but there are occasional exceptions.

A shooting pain lasting a few seconds is common and means nothing. A sensation of a "catch" at the end of a deep breath is also trivial and does not need attention. Chest wall pain can be demonstrated by pressing a finger on the chest at the spot of discomfort and reproducing or aggravating the pain by this maneuver. Pleurisy gets worse with a deep breath; heart pain does not. When inflammation of the outside covering of the heart (pericarditis) is present, the pain may throb with each heart beat. Ulcer pain burns with an empty stomach and gets better with food; gallbladder pain often becomes more intense after a meal. Each of these last four conditions, when suspected, should be evaluated by a physician.

Spasm of the esophagus (gullet) can cause severe pain mimicking a heart attack and is quite different from the acid-burning that we call heartburn. This spasm pain feels as if it is expanding from inside the chest rather than squeezing from the outside as does heart pain. And it is often relieved by a drink of water, while heart pain is not.

When to See the Doctor for Chest Pain

- *Chest pain associated with shortness of breath.*
- *Chest pain associated with irregular pulse.*
- *Chest pain associated with sweating or dizziness.*
- *Chest pain that is severe and lasts more than one-half hour.*
- *Crushing pain beneath the breast bone.*

HOME TREATMENT

If your chest pain is a new sensation and you are not sure what is going on, you should be evaluated promptly in an emergency medical facility. This is a complaint for which it is better to be conservative. See a doctor. Exceptions are chest wall pain, particularly if you had unusual exertion a day or so before, or pain that you are sure is coming from the esophagus. These you can treat with rest and acetaminophen in the case of chest wall pain, and water and antacids in the case of pain coming from the esophagus.

WHAT TO EXPECT AT THE EMERGENCY ROOM

Try to relax on your way to the emergency room. Only about one-quarter of such emergency room visits actually prove to be heart attacks. Once more, if you aren't short of breath, dizzy, or having an irregular pulse, the outlook is very good for you even if you do have a heart attack. So try to relax as much as possible, since stress and anxiety make the problem worse.

If the first few questions after your arrival at the emergency room suggest to the doctor that you may have had a heart attack, many things will happen at once. An electrocardiogram will be taken, and you may be hooked up to a monitor that gives a continuous electrocardiogram. Catheters (tubes) will be placed in your veins to draw blood and give medication. If the electrocardiogram shows that you may have had a heart attack, you are likely to be taken to a coronary care unit, which is a specialized area to care for patients with possible heart attacks. Medication may be given to attempt to dissolve the clot, or a catheter may be passed through the clot to open the artery again. Emergency bypass surgery is now required less frequently because of these newer techniques. In general, be sure to get a second opinion before agreeing to bypass surgery since these operations only help particular kinds of coronary artery disease. Even if the electrocardiogram doesn't show a heart attack, you may still have had one. Blood tests will be taken every few hours to determine if there has been any damage to the heart muscle. If there is no damage, you will be said to have "ruled out" and home you go.

20/ *Shortness of Breath*

This symptom is normal, of course, under circumstances of strenuous activity. The medical term "shortness of breath" does not refer to shortness of breath after heavy exertion, being "breathless" with excitement, or having clogged nasal passages. These innocent instances are not cause for alarm.

On the other hand, when you get "winded" after slight exertion or at rest, wake up in the night out of breath, or have to sleep propped up on several pillows to avoid becoming short of breath, you have a serious problem that should be promptly evaluated by your physician. This can be a sign of heart failure.

If wheezing is present, the problem may be asthma or early emphysema, and again you need the attention of your physician.

If fever is present or if you are coughing up phlegm or pus from your lungs, you may have an infection such as pneumonia, pneumonitis, or bronchitis. Again, you need the doctor.

If shortness of breath comes on suddenly while you are eating, it is likely that food has become lodged in the top of your trachea. Here you need to bend over and get some whacks on the back, and if someone trained is present you should have a Heimlich maneuver performed. (If you don't know exactly what a Heimlich maneuver is, you shouldn't try it.) You can lean over the back of a chair and whack yourself on the back if no one else is around.

If chest pain is present at the same time as shortness of breath, the possibility of heart attack is present, and you need a doctor.

HOME TREATMENT

Rest, relax, and go see the doctor at the emergency room. The problem of shortness of breath is always potentially serious and there isn't much that you can do for this problem at home. If you have had this problem before, sometimes you don't need a visit, but you do need to follow your doctor's advice for what you should be doing under such circumstances.

When to See the Doctor for Shortness of Breath

- *Shortness of breath at rest.*
- *Shortness of breath associated with wheezing.*
- *Shortness of breath occurring suddenly with meals.*
- *Shortness of breath associated with fever.*
- *Persistent shortness of breath of any type.*

WHAT TO EXPECT AT THE DOCTOR'S OFFICE

The physician will thoroughly examine the lungs, heart, and upper airway passages. Often, electrocardiograms (EKG), chest x-rays, and blood tests will be necessary. Depending on the cause and the severity of the problem, hospitalization, fluid pills, heart pills, or asthma medications may be needed. Oxygen is less frequently helpful than commonly imagined and can be hazardous for patients with emphysema; nevertheless, it may be required.

21/ *Irregular Heart Rhythm or Palpitations*

Everyone experiences palpitations, the sensation of your heart beating extremely forcefully, just before you are going to sleep or at a time of strenuous exercise or intense emotion. This is due to a discharge of adrenaline from the adrenal glands. Palpitations are not a serious medical concern, but should be mentioned at your next visit to the doctor. Most people who complain of palpitations do not have heart disease but are overly concerned about the possibility of such disease and thus overly sensitive to normal heart actions. Often this is because of heart disease in parents, other relatives, or friends.

An irregular or very fast pulse may be more serious. There is a normal variation in the pulse with respiration (faster when breathing in, slower when breathing out). Even though the pulse may speed or slow, the normal pulse has a regular rhythm. Occasional extra heart beats occur in nearly everyone. The heart feels as if it is making a "flip-flop." A few of these are normal, but if you are having them five times a minute or more this is a sign to see the doctor. Similarly, if the heart is turning flip-flops two, three, or four times in a row, you should see the doctor.

Sometimes, the heart will change from its normal rhythm quite suddenly into a very rapid rhythm. It may be regular or irregular, but it is going more than 120 times a minute. Any heart rate greater than 120 beats a minute without exercise is cause to check with your physician. Since this problem may have gone back to normal in a few minutes, you may not need to see the doctor right away, but if the rapid rate persists, an immediate visit is indicated.

You should learn to take your own pulse. The pulse can be felt on the inside of the wrist, on one side of the neck, or over the heart itself. Ask the nurse on your next visit to check your method of taking pulses. Take your own pulse and those of your family, noting the variation with respiration. You have to know what normal is before you can readily detect what is abnormal in yourself or others.

HOME TREATMENT

Irregular or rapid cardiac rhythms are a problem for the doctor's office or emergency room. The most frequent causes of rapid heart beat, however, are exercise, anxiety, and fever. Here you may not need the help of a physician. Remember, in doubt, you can always discuss the problem with a physician by phone.

WHAT TO EXPECT AT THE DOCTOR'S OFFICE

Tell the doctor the exact rate of the pulse and whether or not the rhythm was regular. Usually the symptoms will have disappeared by the time you see the doctor, so the accuracy of your story becomes crucial. The doctor will examine your heart and lungs. An electrocardiogram (EKG) may be taken, but it is unlikely to help if the problem is not present when it is being

When to See the Doctor for Irregular Heart Beat

- *Heart turns several flip-flops in a row.*
- *Heart turns flip-flops several times each minute.*
- *Chest pain, dizziness, or shortness of breath are present.*
- *You have episodes of extremely rapid heart rate, regular or irregular, without obvious cause.*

done. A chest x-ray is seldom needed. Do not expect reassurance from a physician that your heart will be sound for the next month, year, or decade. Your doctor has no crystal ball, nor can he or she perform an annual tune-up or oil change. You, not the doctor, are in charge of preventive maintenance of your heart.

22/ *Ankle Swelling*

Swelling of the ankles is a common problem, and the swelling usually affects both legs and may extend up the calves or even the thighs. This is sometimes a heart problem, although more commonly it relates to local problems in the veins. Usually the problem is fluid accumulation, which is most pronounced in the lower legs because of the effects of gravity. If there is excess fluid and you press firmly with your thumb on the area that is swollen, it will squeeze the fluid out of that area and leave a deep impression that will stay for a few moments.

Fortunately, most swelling is due to local causes. Often, breakdowns in the veins over time have made it difficult for blood to be returned to the heart fast enough. This increases pressure in the capillaries and causes fluid to leak out into the tissues, which causes the leg swelling. Swelling is a frequent result of "varicose veins," but it can happen with problems with the deeper veins that are not as obvious. If just one leg is swollen and there is pain and redness, thrombophlebitis may be present and the doctor is needed.

Accumulation of fluid in the body as a result of heart failure can also result in swelling of the ankles. With serious lung disease, such as emphysema, blood may "back up" through the heart and increase pressure in the veins, thus causing swelling of the ankles. More rarely, a problem with the kidneys can result in swelling of the ankles. With serious liver disease, retention of fluid is very common, and this fluid tends to accumulate primarily in the abdomen but is also frequently present in the legs.

HOME TREATMENT

If there is an associated medical problem, the most important treatment will come from your doctor. However, all kinds of ankle swelling can be helped by things that you can do yourself. First, you need to exercise your legs. As you work the muscles, the fluid tends to work back into the veins and lymphatic channels and the swelling tends to go down. Ankle swelling is almost always a signal that your body has too much salt in it. A low-salt diet helps decrease the fluid retention and the ankle swelling.

Elevating your legs can help the fluid drain back into more proper parts of your circulatory system. Lie down and prop your legs up so they are higher than your heart as you rest. One or two pillows under the calves will help. Be sure not to place anything directly under the knees and don't have any constricting clothing or garters on the upper legs. Avoid sitting or standing without moving for long periods of time. If you must be in these positions, work the muscles in your calves by wiggling your feet and toes frequently. Support stockings, by applying constant external pressure, help to reduce ankle swelling.

WHAT TO EXPECT IN THE DOCTOR'S OFFICE

The doctor will conduct a thorough examination including examining the

When to See the Doctor for Ankle Swelling

- *Ankle swelling associated with weight gain of ten pounds or more.*
- *Ankle swelling with an associated medical problem.*
- *Ankle swelling associated with shortness of breath.*
- *Ankle swelling that is painful and involves only one side.*

heart and lungs as well as the legs. Blood tests may be taken to check the function of your kidneys, your liver, and to measure the proteins in your blood. The specific treatment will be directed at whatever underlying cause is found. Diuretics (fluid pills) may be prescribed. These are very effective, but of course they have some side effects. If home treatment is successful, it is generally better than use of drugs.

23/ *Wheezing*

When we breathe in and out, the air must pass through relatively narrow breathing tubes. The largest tubes, the trachea and the main bronchi, are kept open by rings of cartilage that help them hold their shape. However, the smaller ones have muscular walls and are quite flexible. Normally, when we breathe, the power to take air in is provided by our diaphragm, and when we exhale, we do so by relaxing the diaphragm. If there is obstruction in the small breathing tubes, we breathe in pretty much the same but passive relaxation is not enough to help us breathe out. So we have to force the air out, and this takes energy and makes the audible wheeze.

There are two main causes of wheezing—asthma and chronic obstructive pulmonary disease (emphysema). Asthma is most common in young people, and chronic obstructive pulmonary disease in older folks. Asthma can precede and contribute to the development of chronic obstructive pulmonary disease, which is a very severe condition. Asthmatic attacks are frightening but can usually be treated effectively or will go away by themselves. Once permanent chronic damage has occurred, the problem is much more severe and much more difficult to treat. The most important reason for treating reversible episodes of wheezing is to prevent development of chronic obstructive pulmonary disease or emphysema, discussed in the next section. In this section we talk about wheezing caused by spasm of the muscles in the small breathing tubes, with temporary and reversible obstruction.

HOME TREATMENT

You must stop smoking!
You must stop smoking!
You must stop smoking!

Very serious consequences are likely if you don't stop smoking. You could die. You will suffer slow suffocation over many years. Your activities will be limited. You will spend a lot of time in the hospital.

If allergies appear to be contributing to episodes of wheezing, methods of purifying the air are helpful. Air conditioners can be good. A vaporizer that keeps moisture content high is useful. A good fluid intake can help.

When to See the Doctor for Wheezing

- *Rapid onset of severe shortness of breath not immediately responsive to home treatment.*
- *Repeated and frequent episodes of wheezing.*
- *Fever and cough productive of pus or yellow phlegm.*

WHAT TO EXPECT AT THE DOCTOR'S OFFICE

Acute episodes of wheezing are usually treated with adrenaline or similar drugs, aminophylline and its relatives, and sometimes with tranquilizers if anxiety is prominent. Oxygen is usually not helpful nor required.

With repeated attacks, particularly if there is fever or a productive cough, antibiotics may be given. If allergies appear likely and the episodes are seasonal, desensitization procedures can be very helpful. Corticosteroids (prednisone) are effective but can lead to severe long-term side effects if they are continued for very long.

24/ *Emphysema*

Chronic obstructive pulmonary disease (COPD or emphysema) is almost exclusively a disease of smokers. There are rare forms that are genetic or due to other causes. Normally the inner surfaces of the small breathing tubes are kept clear of debris by small moving hairs that propel a thin layer of mucus (with the foreign debris stuck in it) up through the trachea where it is swallowed. Smoking destroys this system of moving hairs so that debris cannot be cleared. As a result, there are frequent and almost continual minor infections, and these obstruct the breathing tubes and cause wheezing. The increased effort and pressure of breathing out, together with the infection, cause a breakdown of the tiny compartments (alveoli) with which we breathe. Normally our lungs have about an *acre* of surface area across which to exchange oxygen and carbon dioxide, because there are many, many small compartments that combine to give a very large surface area. As the walls between the compartments break down, the surface area for gas exchange is greatly decreased and soon the body can't get enough oxygen nor can it get rid of enough carbon dioxide.

Chronic obstructive pulmonary disease is better prevented than treated. Once the hair cells have been destroyed, they don't come back. Once the walls of the small aveoli have broken down, they cannot repair themselves. Primary prevention is to stop smoking or never to start. Secondary prevention is to stop smoking early, before irreversible damage has occurred.

HOME TREATMENT

You have to stop smoking! Chronic obstructive pulmonary disease is the most miserable chronic disease that I know; many people slowly suffocate over a period of 10 or 20 years. You have to do everything you can to arrest the progression, at whatever stage. The central key is to stop cigarette smoking. Weight loss can help, since it decreases the body's need for oxygen. A vaporizer to keep moisture in the air can help your body clear mucus and foreign particles from the lungs. Drinking plenty of fluids can do the same thing. And of course you want to adhere closely to your medical regimen. You need a good doctor.

WHAT TO EXPECT AT THE DOCTOR'S OFFICE

Many medications are helpful, in part. Many of these, such as adrenaline, aminophylline, and inhalants, are the same agents used in asthma, but they are not as effective once chronic structural changes have occurred. Antibiotics are frequently required to decrease problems from constant minor and major infections. Corticosteroids (prednisone) are used by some doctors. I personally like to be very cautious with prednisone-type drugs since they both weaken the tissues and weaken resistance to infection.

Oxygen may be necessary, and low-flow home oxygen is eventually needed by

When to See the Doctor with Emphysema

- *Acute worsening of shortness of breath.*
- *Fever and production of green or yellow phlegm.*
- *Chest pain.*
- *Shortness of breath at rest.*
- *You haven't seen the doctor in three months.*

many patients. Oxygen must be used cautiously and with careful attention to your doctor's advice; too much oxygen can actually shut down your breathing mechanisms and make you worse. Hospitalizations are frequently required as the disease progresses. Cutting a hole in the trachea (tracheostomy) to allow better breathing, together with use of respirators, is sometimes required for emergency treatment.

25/ *Heartburn*

Heartburn is due to irritation of the esophagus, the tube that leads from the mouth to the stomach. The stomach lining is usually protected from the effects of its own acid, but certain factors, such as smoking, caffeine, aspirin, and stress can cause this protection to be lost and for gastritis to occur. The esophagus is not protected against acid, and a back flow of acid from the stomach into the esophagus causes acid irritation. You can often actually feel the acid wash up the esophagus and notice the sour and stinging taste in your mouth. A hiatal hernia aggravates the problem.

Heartburn episodes tend to increase in frequency and severity as we get older. Normally, there is a valve between the stomach and the esophagus that keeps the stomach acid where it should be and prevents it from regurgitating upward. If the acid does go up a little, the swallowing wave that continually goes down through the esophagus carries the acid back down to the stomach where it belongs. The valve is situated right at the diaphragm, and constriction of the diaphragm muscle also helps keep the valve closed. As we age, several of these mechanisms don't work as well. The swallowing wave is somewhat weaker. The valve itself doesn't close as tightly. Often there has been some widening of the space in the diaphragm so that part of the stomach actually goes above the diaphragm (hiatus hernia) and the diaphragm cannot help keep the valve closed. Heartburn by itself is an uncomfortable rather than a severe problem. Home treatment will usually help quite a bit.

HOME TREATMENT

Avoid substances that aggravate the problem. The most common irritants are coffee, tea, alcohol, aspirin, and more recently ibuprofen. The contribution of smoking or stress must be considered. Relief is often obtained with a frequent (every one or two hours) use of nonabsorbable antacids like Maalox, Mylanta, or Gelusil. Antacids should be used with caution by people with heart disease or high blood pressure because of their high salt content. Sodium bicarbonate or Alka-Selzer may give quick relief but is not suitable for frequent use. Low-fat milk may be substituted for antacid, but it adds calories.

If your heartburn episodes occur at night when you are lying down, then you need to get gravity to help you rather than hurt you. Measures that help prevent the back flow of acids from the stomach into the esophagus should be employed: Avoid reclining for at least two hours after eating. Elevate the head of the bed with four-inch to six-inch blocks. Discontinue wearing tight-fitting clothes (girdles, etc.) if applicable. Weight loss helps decrease the pressure on the stomach. If the problem lasts for more than three days, call your doctor.

WHAT TO EXPECT AT THE DOCTOR'S OFFICE

The physician will determine if the problem is due to stomach acid (a peptic acid syndrome). If so, treatment

When to See the Doctor for Heartburn

- *Vomiting of black or bloody material.*
- *Passage of tarlike, black stools when you are not taking iron tablets.*
- *Persistent heartburn pain.*
- *Pain that you think might be heartburn but does not have the characteristics of burning pain just below breast bone or ribs or relief obtained with milk or bland food.*

will be similar to that described under "Home Treatment." Medications to reduce secretion of acid, such as cimetidine, may be prescribed. X-rays of the stomach after swallowing barium (upper GI series) may be done to determine the presence of ulcers and to note if back flow of acid from the stomach into the esophagus is present. Since the treatment for any acid syndrome is essentially the same, an x-ray is usually not done on the first visit. Any indication of bleeding, of course, will require a more vigorous approach to treatment.

26/ *Nausea*

In younger people, nausea is most frequently due to a viral infection. In older people, by far the most frequent reason for nausea is side effects from medications. Once in a while nausea is caused by intolerance to particular foods. Persistent nausea, if it is not related to drugs, can be a sign of a serious problem such as infection, cancer, or scarring at the end of the stomach from ulcers.

Nausea is a warning sign from our stomach that something is wrong and that it is irritated or overfull. It is a signal to us that the vomiting reflex may be triggered, and vomiting brings along an additional set of problems that we would like to avoid if possible.

HOME TREATMENT

The most frequent cause of nausea is aspirin, ibuprofen, or other over-the-counter medications. You started the over-the-counter medication by yourself, and you can stop it by yourself, without a doctor's advice. If you suspect a particular food or spice, of course you will want to avoid it. The remainder of home treatment consists of dealing carefully with the nausea so that it doesn't develop into vomiting. This includes taking your food in frequent small feedings so as not to overload the stomach at any one time, emphasizing fluid intake rather than solid foods, and selecting bland foods such as toast or applesauce.

Alcohol can be a real contributor to nausea, and it aggravates the effects of most of the drugs that irritate the stomach. If alcohol is involved, this is a serious warning sign about your drinking. You will want to avoid alcohol, at least until this problem is over. Smoking tends to aggravate nausea, and it slows the healing of the irritation in the stomach.

WHAT TO EXPECT AT THE DOCTOR'S OFFICE

Almost any prescribed drug can cause nausea. The most frequent offenders are the nonsteroidal, antiinflammatory agents such as piroxicam, naproxen, ibuprofen, ketoprofen, sulindac, and others. Digitalis, blood pressure medications, and antidepressants are other frequent causes. The attentive doctor will review your entire medication schedule and will remove any drugs that are not medically required at this time. If the nausea has been persistent, the history and physical examination will be directed at trying to identify any underlying causes that might be present.

When to See the Doctor for Nausea

- *Nausea possibly due to prescribed medication (call).*
- *Nausea associated with weight loss.*
- *Nausea associated with severe vomiting (see Problem 27).*
- *Nausea persisting more than two weeks.*

Drugs to decrease stomach acid or to coat the stomach may be recommended. In general, antinausea drugs will not be prescribed unless the cause of the nausea is known and can't be avoided. Generally it is not a good idea to use a drug to cover up the side effects caused by another drug.

27/ *Vomiting*

Vomiting in seniors is caused more frequently by medications than by any other cause. Viral infection is another common cause, as is ulcer scarring at the outlet to the stomach, which prevents the stomach from emptying in a timely manner. Alcohol, particularly hard liquor, is another frequent cause. Vomiting is the ultimate complaint that your stomach can make to you. Most of the time vomiting means that the stomach is irritated, has something in it that it doesn't like, or is unable to empty efficiently. Vomiting can also be caused by "central" mechanisms, in which the stomach is all right but the brain is signaling the need to vomit. Drugs can act to cause vomiting either through the central mechanism or by the local irritation mechanism.

A real threat with vomiting is that of dehydration. You can also "aspirate," getting some of the vomitus into the breathing tubes. The speed with which dehydration develops depends on the size of the individual and the frequency of the vomiting. Signs of dehydration include marked thirst, infrequent urination or dark yellow urine, dry mouth, or eyes that appear sunken, and a loss of the normal elasticity of the skin. To determine elasticity, gently pinch the skin on the stomach. When you release it, it should spring back immediately; compare your reaction with another person's skin if necessary. When the skin remains tented up and does not spring back normally, this suggests dehydration.

In addition to dehydration, bleeding (black or bloody vomitus) or severe abdominal pain requires the physician's attention immediately. Some abdominal discomfort accompanies almost every case of vomiting, but severe pain is unusual unless the problem is potentially serious.

HOME TREATMENT

The objective of home treatment is to provide as much fluid as possible without upsetting the stomach any further. Sip clear fluids such as water or ginger ale. Suck on ice chips if nothing else will stay down. Don't drink very much at any one time, and avoid solid foods until you are sure that you can keep the liquids down. If fever is present, it will increase your need for fluid, so take in as much as possible. As your condition improves, add soups, bouillion, jello, toast, and applesauce. Work up slowly to a normal diet. If you have questions, call your physician.

WHAT TO EXPECT AT THE DOCTOR'S OFFICE

The history and physical examination will be focused on determining the existence of any dehydration as well as the possible causes of the vomiting. Drugs should always be the first suspects. Vomiting can be caused by almost any medication on occasion, but the most frequent offenders are those that notoriously affect the stomach, such as aspirin or nonsteroidal, antiinflammatory drugs such as piroxicam, sulindac, naproxen, ibuprofen, or indomethacin. The doctor should review your medication schedule

When to See the Doctor for Vomiting

- *Black or bloody vomitus.*
- *Severe abdominal pain.*
- *Vomiting following a head injury.*
- *Unable to retain any fluids for 12 hours or more.*
- *Vomiting associated with fever or very hot weather.*
- *Vomiting in a diabetic patient.*
- *Persistence of vomiting for more than two days.*

in detail and will probably want to suspend treatment with anything that is not absolutely essential. (An essential medication may have to be given by injection or by vein if you can't keep anything down.) Blood tests and a urinalysis may be ordered but are not always necessary. Plain x-rays of the abdomen are usually not very helpful, but special x-ray procedures may be necessary in some cases. If dehydration is present, intravenous fluids may be given either in the doctor's office or in the hospital. Antivomiting drugs are often *not* a good thing to use, since they just cover up the problem.

28/ *Diarrhea*

Diarrhea is a defense mechanism the body uses to quickly get rid of toxic substances, viruses, and bacteria. Viral infections are the most common cause, although in seniors prescribed medications come in a close second. Dehydration and bleeding are the greatest risks. With a viral illness, diarrhea is often accompanied by nausea and vomiting, headaches, and other aches and pains. Bacterial infections can produce diarrhea or dysentery, and sometimes antibiotics are required. Black or bloody diarrhea may be a signal of significant bleeding from the stomach or intestine. However, medications containing iron or bismuth (Pepto Bismol) may also turn the stool black.

Cramping, intermittent, gaslike pains are usual with diarrhea, but severe steady abdominal pain is not. Bleeding or severe abdominal pain requires the immediate attention of the physician. If you suspect a medication, you will want to call the prescribing physician and ask what to do.

HOME TREATMENT

As with vomiting, the major objective in treating diarrhea is to take in as much fluid as possible without upsetting the intestinal tract any further. Sip clear fluids such as water or ginger ale. If nothing else will stay down, sucking on ice chips is usually tolerated and provides some fluid. When clear fluids are tolerated easily, you can start with food again. Relatively constipating foods such as bananas, rice, applesauce, and toast should be added back first. Milk and fats should generally be avoided for several days.

Nonprescription drugs are relatively infrequent causes, although prescription medicines frequently cause diarrhea. If you suspect that an over-the-counter drug is responsible, you will want to stop it. In general, we think that you should not take an antidiarrhea medication without at least calling your doctor first.

WHAT TO EXPECT AT THE DOCTOR'S OFFICE

The thorough history and physical examination with special attention to assessing dehydration will be done. The abdomen will be examined. Frequently the stools will be examined under the microscope, and occasionally a culture will be taken. A urine specimen may be examined to assist in assessing dehydration. In the case of a bacterial infection, an antibiotic may be used.

Current medical thinking is moving away from deliberately stopping diarrhea by use of Kaopectate, Lomotil, or other drugs since these may delay the elimination of toxic substances from the body through the diarrhea mechanism, and they just cover up the problem. Still, they can help prevent dehydration and are sometimes needed.

Chronic diarrhea may require a more extensive stool evaluation, blood tests, and sometimes x-ray examination of the intestinal tract. As with vomiting, severe dehydration will require intravenous fluids; this may be done in the doctor's office or may require hospitalization.

When to See the Doctor for Diarrhea

- *Black or bloody stools.*
- *Severe abdominal pain.*
- *Infrequent urination, dry skin and mouth, and other signs of dehydration.*
- *Diarrhea with fever, vomiting, or in hot weather lasting more than a day.*
- *Severe diarrhea lasting more than three days.*
- *Mild diarrhea lasting more than two weeks.*

The physician will review your medication schedule, with particular attention to the prime offenders such as meclofenemate (Meclomen), auranofin (Ridaura), and other drugs used for arthritis and musculoskeletal pain. Most antibiotics, after several days' treatment, can also result in diarrhea. Almost any drug can cause diarrhea on occasion, however, so all will be suspect.

29/ *Constipation*

Many people are preoccupied with their bowel movements. Concern about the shape of the stool, its consistency, its color, and the frequency of bowel movements is often reported to physicians, and usually such complaints are medically trivial. Only rarely, and then usually in seniors, does a change in bowel habits signal a serious problem. Weight loss and thin, pencil-like stool suggest a tumor of the lower bowel. Abdominal pain and a swollen abdomen suggest a possible bowel obstruction. Again, medications or an unhealthy diet are frequent contributors.

HOME TREATMENT

We like to encourage a healthy diet for the bowel, followed by a healthy disinterest in the details of the stool elimination process. The diet should contain fresh fruits and vegetables for their natural laxative action and for adequate fiber residue. Fiber is present in brans, celery, and whole wheat breads and is absent in foods that have been too completely processed. Fiber draws water into the stool and adds bulk; thus it decreases the transit time from mouth to bowel movement and softens the stool. It also decreases the effort of elimination.

Bowel movements may occur three times daily or once each three days and still be normal. Stools may change in color, texture, consistency, or bulk without need for concern. Movements may be regular or irregular. Don't worry about them unless there is a major deviation.

If laxatives are required, we prefer Metamucil, which is a fiber and bulk laxative. Milk of Magnesia is satisfactory, but it and stronger traditional laxatives should not be used over a long period. For an acute problem, an enema may help. Fleet's enemas are handy and disposable. If such remedies are needed more than occasionally, ask your doctor about the problem on your next routine visit.

WHAT TO EXPECT AT THE DOCTOR'S OFFICE

Expect a rectal examination and, often, inspection of the lower bowel through a long metal or plastic tube called a sigmoidoscope. An x-ray of the lower bowel (barium enema) is often needed. Sometimes, particularly in a person limited to bed, the stool becomes so impacted that it cannot be excreted. Often in such a case the constipation alternates with diarrhea or fecal soiling (incontinence). The doctor can break up the stool and then use enemas so that the way is clear again. If you have a "fecal impaction" it can make you feel generally ill, with fever, nausea, and other problems. Releasing a fecal impaction can be one of the minor miracles of medical treatment. If you have only a minor constipation problem you will probably receive advice from your doctor similar to that given above under "Home Treatment,"

When to See the Doctor for Constipation

- *Constipation associated with thin, pencil-like stools.*
- *Constipation associated with abdominal pain and bloating.*
- *Constipation associated with weight loss of more than five pounds.*
- *Hard stools with frequency less than once each four days.*
- *Constipation alternating with diarrhea or fecal incontinence.*
- *Persistence of constipation to the next routine doctor visit.*

without examination or procedures. Remember that we do recommend a rectal examination each year as screening for rectal cancers, and if you have a complaint of minor constipation, it should remind you and your doctor that you need this examination.

30/ *Abdominal Pain*

Abdominal pain can be a sign of a serious condition. Fortunately, minor causes for these symptoms are much more frequent than major ones.

Abdominal pain can come from the esophagus, the stomach, the bowel, the female organs, the rectum, the gallbladder, an outpouching of the bowel, or from other organs. Appendix pain usually occurs in the right lower quarter, kidney pain involves the back, the gallbladder involves the right upper quarter, the stomach the upper abdomen, and the bladder, colon, or female organs the lower areas. Exceptions to these rules do occur. Pain from hollow organs such as the bowel or gallbladder tends to be intermittent and to resemble gas pains or colic. Pain from solid organs such as the kidneys, spleen, or liver tends to be more constant. There are exceptions to these rules also.

In seniors, the colon is more frequently a source of pain than earlier in life. Colon out-pouchings, called diverticuli, can become inflamed just like the appendix and cause "diverticulitis." Minor (or even major) obstruction of the colon is not uncommon.

If pain is very severe or bleeding from the bowel occurs, obviously you need to see a physician immediately. Pain localized to one area is more suggestive of a serious problem than generalized pain, although again there are many exceptions to this rule.

Gas pains and minor viral infections are the easy ones. These usually respond to home treatment.

HOME TREATMENT

If the pain eventually proves to be due to a serious problem, the stomach should be empty to allow prompt surgery or diagnostic tests. So anticipate this possibility. Sips of water or other clear fluids may be taken, but avoid solid foods. A bowel movement, passage of gas through the rectum, or a good belch may give relief—don't hold back. If you haven't had a bowel movement for several days, an enema can sometimes give relief. Be gentle. A warm bath helps some patients. The key to home treatment is periodic reevaluation. Any persistent pain should be evaluated at the emergency room or the physician's office. Home treatment should be reserved for mild pains that resolve within 24 hours or are clearly identifiable as viral gastroenteritis, gas pains, heartburn, or another minor problem.

When to See the Doctor for Abdominal Pain

- *Passage of black or bloody stools.*
- *Very severe abdominal pain.*
- *Abdominal injury in the last 48 hours.*
- *Presence of nausea, vomiting, diarrhea, or fever.*
- *Persistence for more than 24 hours.*

WHAT TO EXPECT AT THE DOCTOR'S OFFICE

The physician will perform a thorough examination, particularly of the abdomen. Usually a white count, urinalysis, and often other laboratory tests will be done. X-rays are often not important with pain of short duration but are sometimes needed. Observation in the hospital may be required. If the initial evaluation was negative but pain persists, reevaluation is necessary, and the physician may want to check up on you daily or even twice a day.

31/ *Rectal Pain*

Rectal pain relatively seldom indicates a major medical problem, but the discomfort may materially interfere with the quality of life. Unlike some other medical problems, rectal pain does not yield the dividend of a good topic for social conversation.

Hemorrhoids (piles) are the most common cause of these symptoms. There is a network of veins around the anus, both inside and outside the rectal opening. These veins tend to enlarge with age, particularly in overweight individuals who sit a good deal during the day. Straining to have a bowel movement and the passage of hard compacted stools tend to irritate these veins, which may become inflamed, tender, or clogged. Small tears in the rectum may occur. Because of the surrounding colon bacteria, such sores become infected and are slow to heal. The veins themselves are the "hemorrhoids." They may be external to the anal opening and visible, or they may be inside and invisible. Pain and inflammation usually go away within a few days or a few weeks, but this interval can be extremely uncomfortable. After healing, a small flap or tag of vein and scar tissue often remains.

Cancer of the rectum is of course a serious problem, but it is seldom painful; this is why rectal examinations are required to locate these asymptomatic tumors while they are small. A tumor of the rectum can make bowel movements difficult and can make the stools thin and pencil-like, but usually this process is not painful.

Bleeding from the digestive tract should be taken seriously. You don't have to worry so much about bright red, relatively light bleeding seen as blood on the toilet paper that comes directly from hemorrhoids, but blood from higher in the digestive tract (which will be burgundy or black in color) is much more serious. Blood from hemorrhoids will be on the outside of the stool but will not be mixed into the stool substance; such bleeding is not medically significant unless it persists for several weeks.

HOME TREATMENT

Soften the stool by including more fresh fruits and fiber (bran, celery, whole wheat bread) in the diet or by use of fiber bulk (Metamucil). Laxatives such as Milk of Magnesia are sometimes useful but generally are not as good as bulk laxatives and fresh sources of fiber.

Keep the area scrupulously clean. After a bowel movement, take a shower or bath and soap and clean the area around the rectum. After gently drying the painful area, apply zinc oxide paste or powder to protect against further irritation. The various proprietary hemorrhoid preparations are less satisfactory. We prefer not to use compounds with a local anesthetic agent, because these compounds may sensitize and irritate the area and may prolong healing rather than speed it; such compounds usually have a "caine" in the brand name or in the list of ingredients. "Internal" hemorrhoids sometimes may be helped by using a soothing suppository in addition to stool-softening

When to See the Doctor for Rectal Pain

- *Black or burgundy color to stools.*
- *Narrowing or changed consistency of the stools.*
- *Persistence of pain for more than a week despite home treatment.*

measures. If relief is not complete within a week, see the doctor. Even if the problem resolves quickly, mention it to your doctor on your next visit.

WHAT TO EXPECT AT THE DOCTOR'S OFFICE

The doctor will examine the anus and rectum. If a clot is found, the hemorrhoid vein may be lanced and the clot removed. Major hemorrhoid surgery is seldom required and should be reserved for the most persistent problems. Usually you will receive advice similar to that given above under "Home Treatment."

32/ *Incontinence*

We are all born unable to control our bowels and bladders, and as we grow older there is a tendency for some of these problems to return. The subject of incontinence is a large and complicated one since there are many causes and many treatments. Incontinence is not a hopeless condition. The vast majority of people can be greatly helped, and many times the problems can be made to entirely disappear.

As we age, the female uterus and pelvic floor sag, changing the angle at which the urethra exits the body and predisposing to leakage of urine. In men, benign enlargement of the prostate gland tends to block passage of urine from the bladder until finally the bladder must overflow. Infections of the urinary tract can cause an urgency for which there is no time to react. With age, there are sometimes uninhibited contractions of the bladder muscles, resulting in increased pressures at unexpected times. There can be decreased sensitivity to the presence of a full bladder. Once urgency is experienced it can be difficult to get to the toilet in time. Drugs such as diuretics can cause major surges in urine flow. Other drugs, such as tranquilizers, anticholinergics, antidepressants, and others can block the normal voiding mechanisms, resulting in retention of urine and then incontinence. Stones in the bladder can predispose to infection.

Fecal incontinence is usually due to the presence of impacted stool in the rectum resulting in diarrhea and incontinence around the impacted stool.

Problems with either urinary or fecal incontinence should be reported to your physician. This is not a complaint to be shy about, since if you let it persist, it will begin to affect all parts of your life and even will affect your image of yourself.

HOME TREATMENT

There are many approaches at home that can be of great help, but you should talk with your doctor about which ones are most appropriate for you. For fecal incontinence it is important that your diet contain adequate fiber, water, and bulk. A soft stool passed twice a week is normal, but you should consider hard impacted stool (even if passed in small amounts twice daily) as a problem to be addressed. Fiber, as in whole wheat grains, brans, celery, fresh fruits, and vegetables, is helpful. Metamucil can be used to add bulk. Since the presence of impacted feces in the rectum can make you feel bad all over, it is important to get this relieved immediately. The doctor will help.

Performance of the bladder can often be improved by practice with the muscles that control the urinary outlet. Practice stopping urination in midstream and then starting again. This is often very difficult, especially for women, but the exercise will build stronger sphincter muscles. Deliberately contracting the muscles around your anus and urinary tract for a second or two, then relaxing, then repeating will build strength in these muscles and help tighten the pelvic floor. Many doctors

When to See the Doctor for Incontinence

- *Repeated incontinence of urine, even small amounts.*
- *Incontinence of feces.*

recommend that these exercises be done up to 100 times daily. If you have trouble getting to the toilet on time, consider keeping a urine receptacle close at hand. Always suspect that drugs you are taking might be aggravating the problem; be sure to bring this possibility to the attention of your physician.

The techniques of double-voiding can be helpful. Here, you empty the bladder as much as you can, wait a minute or so, and then empty it again. It is surprising how much additional urine will sometimes be present. "Bladder drill" consists of urinating at fixed intervals, perhaps each four hours, during the day, whether the sensation of urgency is present or not; this can help.

WHAT TO EXPECT AT THE DOCTOR'S OFFICE

The physician will perform a complete examination, with emphasis on the abdomen, rectum, and the urinary openings. Urinalysis will usually be performed. If there are abnormalities, cystoscopy (inspection of the inside of the bladder) may be indicated. The gynecologist and the urologist are the specialists who are most familiar with these problems. If simple treatments don't work, there are a variety of urodynamic studies that can pinpoint the exact problem and lead to more specific treatment. In women, the physician will sometimes prescribe a local estrogen cream, which can be surprisingly effective by softening the tissues and making them more elastic. Uterine or pelvic suspension operations are sometimes needed. Men may require prostectomy. Internal or external (in men) catheters are sometimes necessary.

33/ *Difficulty Voiding in Males*

Paying some attention to the process of urination can tell you a good bit about your general health as well as about specific problems in the urinary tract. At least once a day your urine should be copious and nearly colorless; otherwise, you are probably not drinking enough fluid. Blood in the urine can be a sign of kidney stone or an early sign of a bladder cancer, although sometimes a blood vessel will break spontaneously or during exercise and just bleed for a little bit. Repeated blood in the urine is a clear signal to see the doctor.

Dark golden urine with a yellow foam can be a sign of jaundice; sometimes you can see the signs of liver disease in the urine before you can see the color changes in the skin or white of the eyes.

The most common urinary tract problems in men have to do with the prostate gland. The prostate gland surrounds the urethra and the urine must pass through this gland to get to the outside. Three things can go wrong with the prostate gland: It can become infected, it can gradually enlarge with age (benign prostatic hypertrophy), and it can develop a cancer. Prostatic cancer is very common, but, fortunately, it is usually a very slow growing and localized cancer so there is quite a bit of time to find it, and it relatively seldom results in death. Benign prostatic hypertrophy can require surgery to open up the urethra again. Infection of the prostate gland (or elsewhere in the urinary tract) can be helped by home treatment but may also require antibiotics or prostatic massage.

Prostate problems all result in narrowing of the urethra, the tube that takes urine to the outside. As a result, urine tends to back up behind the obstruction in the bladder, voiding urine requires more pressure of the bladder muscle, the bladder gradually gets stretched and enlarged because of the retained urine, and then the bladder muscle doesn't work as well, and the retained urine is likely to get infected. This whole chain of events follows from the partial obstruction. The first signs are usually hesitancy in starting the urine flow, some dribbling after urination, and some loss of force of the urinary stream.

HOME TREATMENT

Definitive treatment of urinary tract infection requires an antibiotic (which may not alter the symptoms for 24 hours). Quicker relief is afforded by home treatment, which should be started immediately, even if you are taking an antibiotic. Drink lots of fluids. Increase fluid intake to the maximum you can tolerate, up to several gallons of fluid in the first 24 hours. Bacteria are literally washed from the body during the resulting copious urination. Drink fruit juices, since they put more acid into the urine. Cranberry juice is the most effective, as it contains a natural antibiotic, mandelic acid.

Except for these measures, there isn't too much home treatment available. You usually need a doctor for these symptoms.

When to See the Doctor for Difficulty Voiding

- *Urinary symptoms associated with vomiting, back pain, or shaking chills.*
- *Discharge from the penis.*
- *Hesitancy, dribbling, or weak urinary stream.*
- *Blood in the urine.*
- *Persistent symptoms for two weeks.*

WHAT TO EXPECT AT THE DOCTOR'S OFFICE

A urinalysis and culture will be performed. A rectal examination will be performed with particular emphasis on feeling the prostate gland. Massage of this gland can frequently milk an infection out and relieve symptoms quite dramatically. If infection is suspected, an antibiotic will be prescribed. With symptoms of hesitancy, dribbling, or weak stream, the urethra may be visualized through a cystoscope and the bladder mechanics measured by special procedures performed by a urologist. Sometimes the narrow passage may be widened just by using a dilating instrument called a "sound," but frequently surgery is required. Transurethral resection of the prostate (opening the channel by surgery performed through the urethra without an external incision) is one of the most common operations performed and is usually successful in relieving obstruction.

34/ *Difficult or Painful Voiding in Females*

The best-known symptoms of bladder infection are pain and burning on urination, frequent and urgent urination, and blood in the urine. These symptoms are not always caused by infection due to bacteria, although this is the most frequent cause. They can be due to a viral infection, excessive use of caffeine-containing beverages, bladder spasm, ingestion of some peppers and spices, or they can occur without an obvious cause.

Bladder infection is much more common in women than it is in men; most women have it at one time or another. The female urethra, the tube leading from the bladder to the outside of the body, is only about one-half inch long, a very short distance for bacteria to travel to reach the bladder. The bacteria usually come from the area around the rectum, also only a short distance away.

Vomiting, back pain, or teeth-chattering, body-shaking chills are not typical of bladder infections and suggest that an infection may have moved to the kidneys. This is more serious and requires more vigorous treatment and follow-up.

Some physicians have developed procedures by which a patient with these symptoms can obtain a urinalysis without first seeing the physician. If the urinalysis indicates a possible bacterial infection, the patient is seen and appropriate therapy begun. If this is not the case, the patient is directed to use home treatment for 24 hours. If there is no relief during that time, the patient is then seen.

Many bacterial bladder infections will respond to home treatment alone, although the cure may not be complete. Bacteria double in numbers as frequently as every 20 minutes. Yet, if you void completely, you may excrete 99 percent of the bacteria in the bladder into the toilet. If your urine flow is fast enough, you can wash out superficial bladder infections.

Still, it makes good sense to use antibiotics when appropriate, and this has become standard medical practice. Antibiotics may be especially important in recurrent bladder infections. Even if you are inclined toward doing without drugs, you should see the doctor for these symptoms unless they respond quickly and completely to home treatment.

HOME TREATMENT

Definitive treatment of urinary tract infection requires an antibiotic. Quicker relief is afforded by home treatment, which should be started immediately. Drink a lot of fluids. Increase fluid intake up to the maximum you can tolerate, and this can include several *gallons* of fluid in the first 24 hours. Drink fruit juices; putting more acid into the urine, while less important than the quantity of fluids, may help bring relief. Cranberry juice is the most effective, as it contains a natural antibiotic, mandelic acid.

Begin home treatment as soon as symptoms are noted. For women with recurrent

When to See the Doctor for Painful Voiding

- *Urinary symptoms associated with vomiting, back pain, or shaking chills.*
- *The problem is associated with a new, irritating vaginal discharge.*
- *Problems are extremely severe and painful.*
- *Symptoms have persisted for 48 hours despite home treatment.*

problems, an important preventive measure is to wipe the toilet tissue from front to back (not back to front) following urination and defecation.

WHAT TO EXPECT AT THE DOCTOR'S OFFICE

A urinalysis and culture should be performed. The back and abdomen are usually examined. If a discharge is present, an examination of both the vagina and the discharge is often necessary. With preexisting kidney disease or recurrent infections a more detailed history and physical exam are needed and extra laboratory studies may be necessary.

If urinary tract infection is proved, an antibiotic should be prescribed. Sulfa drugs and ampicillin are the most commonly used unless there is an allergy to them.

35/ *Breast Examination*

There are three parts to the breast examination: self-examination, the physician examination, and mammography. To minimize your chances of breast cancer, you need all three.

Most lumps in the breast are not cancer. Most women will have a lump in a breast at some time during their life. Many women's breasts are naturally lumpy (benign fibrocystic disease). Obviously every lump or possible lump cannot and should not be subjected to surgery.

There are advantages of each of the three techniques for early detection of cancers, and that is why you need all of them. If breast self-examination is practiced regularly, it is the most important single technique. You know your breasts and are the best observer to spot anything unusual. Moreover, you can do this procedure monthly or even more often, and this gives a better chance that a cancer can be picked up while it is very small. The physician examination will very seldom pick up a lump that you didn't know was there. (Often the physician will have to have the patient locate a suspect lump so that it can be examined.) But the physician does know what cancer feels like and which lumps should be biopsied and which not.

Mammography is an x-ray technique for visualizing suspect lumps in the breast. It can find lumps that you can't feel, especially in large-breasted women or women with preexisting fibrocystic disease that renders self-examination or physician examination more difficult. Essentially all doctors agree that mammography should be performed yearly in women over the age of 50. It is not enough by itself, however, since it is not impossible for a cancer to begin the month after one mammogram and to have become widespread before the next.

HOME EXAMINATION

Breast self-examination should be monthly.

The technique is as follows:

1. Examine your breasts in the mirror, first with your arms at your side and then with both arms over your head. The breasts should look the same. Watch for any change in shape or size or for dimpling of the skin. Occasionally a lump that is difficult to feel will be quite obvious just by looking.

2. Next, while lying flat, examine the left breast using the finger tips of the right hand and pressing the breast tissue against the chest wall. Do not "pinch" the breast tissue between the fingers; all breast tissue feels a bit lumpy when you do this. The left hand should be behind your head while you examine the inner half of the left breast and down at your side when you examine the outer half. Do not neglect the part of the breast immediately underneath the nipple or that which extends outward from the breast toward the under arm. A small pillow under the left shoulder may help.

3. Repeat this process on the opposite side.

When to See the Doctor for Breast Examination

- *Mammography has not been performed for over one year.*
- *Physician breast examination has not been performed in over one year.*

Any lump detected should be brought to the attention of your physician. Regular self-examination will tell you how long it has been present and whether it has changed in size. This information is very helpful in deciding what to do about the lump; even the doctor often has difficulty with this decision. Self-examination is an absolute necessity for a woman with naturally lumpy breasts; the woman is the only one who can really know whether the lump is new, old, or has changed size. For all women, regular self-examination offers the best hope that surgery will be performed when, and only when, it is necessary.

WHAT TO EXPECT AT THE DOCTOR'S OFFICE

The yearly examination should usually be designed to take care of all these little maintenance items at the same time with minimum nuisance and less expense. The physician breast examination, a yearly rectal examination, the gynecological examination, mammography, checking the stool for blood, and if desired an electrocardiogram and sigmoidoscopy can all be done at the same time.

If surgery for breast cancer is recommended, usually the best procedure is a "lumpectomy." If "radical mastectomy" is being considered, with removal of the entire breast and nearby lymph nodes, be sure to get a second opinion before deciding that this is necessary.

36/ *The Gynecologic Examination and the Pap Smear*

Examination of the female reproductive organs, usually called a "pelvic examination," should be performed annually in conjunction with the annual "Pap" smear. The major goal is early cancer detection. The examination can detect cancer of the rectum, of the uterine cervix, of the body of the uterus, and often of the ovaries. Clues may be obtained for bladder or colon tumors as well. These examinations yield a great deal of information and are important. By understanding the phases of the examination and your role in them, you can make it possible for an adequate examination to be done quickly and with a minimum of discomfort.

WHAT TO EXPECT IN THE DOCTOR'S OFFICE

The key word during the gynecologic examination is "relax"; you may hear it several times. The vagina is a muscular organ, and if the muscles are tense, a difficult and uncomfortable examination is inevitable. You may be asked to take several deep breaths in an effort to obtain relaxation.

Usually the best pelvic examinations are done by those who do them most often. You do not necessarily need a gynecologist, but be sure that your internist or family practitioner does "pelvics" on a regular basis before you request a yearly gynecological exam. The nurse practitioner who does pelvic examinations regularly is usually expert. The Pap smear alone does not require a great deal of experience and is the single most important part of the examination. Many physicians will also perform a rectal or recto-vaginal (one finger in rectum and one in vagina) examination. These examinations can provide additional information about problems within the pelvis as well as those in the rectum.

Since the Pap test is of unique importance to women, you should be familiar with the basics of the procedure. A scraping of the cervix and a sample of the vaginal secretions is obtained with the aid of a speculum. This provides cells for study under the microscope. A trained technician (a cytologist) can then classify the cells according to their microscopic characteristics. There are five classes. Classes I and II are negative for tumor cells. Classes III and IV are suspicious but not definite for tumors. Class V is definitely a cancer. If your smear is Class III or Class IV, your physician will ask you to return for another Pap test or a biopsy of the cervix. This does not mean that cancer is definite. If your smear is Class V, your physician will explain the approach to confirming the diagnosis and starting treatment.

Pap smears are an effective tumor-finding test for two reasons. First, a single test detects approximately 90 percent of the most common cancers of the womb (cervical cancer) and 70 to 80 percent

When to See the Doctor for a Gynecologic Exam

- *You have not had a "yearly checkup" in more than a year.*
- *You have a new discharge or bleeding.*

of the second most common (the uterus). Second, both of these common types of cancer usually grow slowly. Current evidence indicates that it often may take 10 years or more for a single focus of cancer in the cervix to spread. Thus there is an excellent chance that regular Pap smears will detect the cancer before it spreads.

37/ *Difficulty Getting Dressed*

The rest of the problem discussions in this section relate to your daily activities. Arthritis can limit your everyday activities, as can heart disease, surgery, neurologic conditions, and other medical problems. These limitations are especially frustrating because we take our ability to perform simple tasks for granted. The frustration sometimes leads to withdrawal rather than to confronting and dealing with the problem.

Usually these problems can be readily helped without professional advice. Developing your own solutions can be a source of real satisfaction. If sickness or frailty is sufficiently severe to affect your daily life, take pride in finding ways to meet the challenge. A few techniques are suggested here, but you will soon learn to invent your own best solutions.

Problems with dressing are usually related to the fine finger movements needed to fasten small buttons, the shoulder action necessary to bring clothes over the head or to fasten garments behind the back, or the difficulty in reaching the feet to put on trousers, shoes, or socks. Other problems come from trouble opening a dresser drawer or getting to the dresser.

HOME TREATMENT

The idea is to make everything as easy as possible. Put the dresser near the bed. Use a dresser of light-weight wood with small, well-lubricated drawers. Replace small knobs with big handles.

Select clothes that are easy to put on. Slip-on shoes, front-fastening garments, zippers with big ring pulls, wrap-around robes, clothes with Velcro fasteners, clip-on ties, stretch belts that hook rather than buckle. Get a friend—or several. Perhaps you have a friend (or spouse) with whom you can exchange tasks, each of you doing what you are good at. A friendly "handyperson" and someone who can use a sewing machine, if you cannot, can be very helpful. Velcro, a marvelous material that sticks to itself simply by applying slight pressure and pulls apart just as easily can be a wonderful replacement for buttons, shoelaces, belts, bra hooks, and other fastenings. You can sew it on everything. The handyperson can make some of the gadgets you may need.

Get or make gadgets. A long-handled shoe horn, garter snaps or spring clothes pins, or a piece of tape for helping to put on socks. A closet hook on the end of a dowel to extend your reach can make life much simpler. Other suggestions include a valet stand to hold your shirt while you put an arm through, a wire button hook for small buttons, and a collar-extender loop to make buttoning that top collar button easier.

WHAT TO EXPECT FROM THE HEALTH PROFESSIONAL

Occupational therapists are trained to help you with this kind of problem. The key word is "adaptive"; the therapist will suggest ways in which you can adapt to your disability. The therapist will also know the sources in your area for

When to See the Health Professional for Difficulty in Dressing

- *Despite home treatment, you are unable to clothe yourself adequately.*
- *Your inability to dress limits your other activities.*

special gadgets and appliances. If you have a long-term arthritis problem or other problems with your musculoskeletal system, look to *The Arthritis Helpbook*, which is available in book stores or through the Arthritis Foundation. It contains many hints, pictures, and sources for materials. See Appendix C for details.

38/ *Using the Toilet*

Dignity is a crucial part of the problem here. We tend to feel uncomfortable asking another person to help us with our eliminations, so this problem very often goes unmentioned. However, with a few fairly simple measures, a lot of difficulty can be avoided.

Remember, the idea is to make necessary daily activities as easy as possible. This is a sensible idea for everybody, of course, but if you have a physical limitation, the defects in the way our society is designed become obvious. What is merely an annoyance for others is a real nuisance to you. And if you can save a few seconds (and some energy) at tasks you must repeat many times, the savings become substantial.

The biggest problem is usually the effort involved in getting on and off of the toilet. Muscle weakness in the legs, contractures in the hips, or arthritis of the knees can act to make getting up and down a problem. We discourage deep knee bends, because they stress the knees too much; the action involved in using the toilet is almost the same.

Patients with severe disability or with arthritis of the wrists sometimes have trouble using toilet paper. And a problem with the bowels, whether it is diarrhea or constipation, can make the whole thing more difficult than it need be.

HOME TREATMENT

You need some physical aids. The most important one is a raised toilet seat. In a major remodeling, you can have toilets installed three to five inches higher than standard, or you can simply purchase a raised seat at a hospital supply store. Don't underestimate the importance of the raised seat; many people have trouble visualizing how much it will help until they have tried it.

An armrest unit can be attached to the toilet bolts and used together with the raised seat. This permits you to use your arms as well as your legs in getting up and down. Alternatively, a safety bar can be installed on the wall. The bar will serve to steady you and to take some of your weight as you stand and sit.

Severely affected persons can use a glider commode to put a toilet in a nearby location, but we don't find too much use for these. Sometimes they encourage a person to be bedbound when he or she could be more active.

For holding toilet paper, your reach can be extended by a variety of different gadgets. You can make tissue holders from knitting needles or coat hangers, or use tongs with plastic tips.

Diarrhea or constipation contributes to the problem of using the toilet, either because of increased frequency or increased straining. So healthy dietary habits (but not obsession with bowel frequency) are important. A good diet should include plenty of fruits and

When to See the Health Professional for Difficulties with the Toilet

- *After home treatment, you still require the assistance of another person in order to use the toilet.*
- *Despite home treatment, the problem is getting worse.*

vegetables as well as bran and whole wheat breads. Exercise regularly and avoid laxatives. If a medication must be taken, use Metamucil—a teaspoonful in a glass of water twice a day; this will increase bulk and stabilize the stool.

WHAT TO EXPECT FROM THE HEALTH PROFESSIONAL

The occupational therapist may well have some additional hints for you and will know the places to purchase anything you may need. The therapist might visit your home; if so, take advantage of this visit to inquire about hints for the other rooms of your house or apartment as well.

The social worker may be able to help you find a source of funds to pay for those things that are too costly for you. Remember that any expenditures you must make to equip your house because of disability are tax deductible; ask your doctor for a prescription for the raised toilet seat, safety bar, or whatever on your next visit; the tax people might want to see it. Your doctor will appreciate your not making a special trip just to obtain such documentation.

39/ *Bathing and Hygiene*

These activities are closely tied into how we feel about ourselves, giving them an importance beyond the medical requirement for decent hygiene. We feel helpless and humiliated if we cannot keep ourselves looking clean or if we must worry about the way we may smell, and these worries may cause us to withdraw from social activities. So these are crucial concerns. The success of other activities may depend on how well we can adapt to problems with bathing, hygiene, and grooming. Some major changes in the home may be necessary for patients with severe disabilities, but the rewards can be dramatic.

Problems usually center around how to get in and out of a tub or shower, how to hold a toothbrush or comb, or how to reach all parts of the body. The modern house is not very well designed for efficient living, and the patient with disability needs to live as efficiently as possible. So you may have to be quite resourceful and do some inventing.

HOME TREATMENT

For the bathtub, mount rails on the wall to help you get in and out safely. Safety rails that mount on the side of the tub are available at hospital supply stores. A suction-cup mat or nonskid tape on the bottom of the tub can help prevent you from slipping. A shower is better for many people, but again use the nonskid tape for safety. A telephone-type shower head that moves up and down on a metal rod often helps. Single-lever faucets are easier to manage than old-fashioned ones that require a strong twist to turn on and keep dripping after you turn them off. Don't use soap dishes or plumbing to support your weight; they can pull out of the wall. A sitting shower is possible if you can't stand for long; use a bath bench with suction cups on the legs. Put the soap in a cloth bag on a string around your neck to eliminate that terrible search for the dropped soap. A shower caddy hanging from the shower head is useful to keep shampoo and brushes close by. A back-scrubbing strap can make that chore easy—and it feels good. A bath mitt can help in scrubbing. To dry off, just put on a terry-cloth robe and let it soak up the water.

Put built-up handles on combs, toothbrushes, and hair brushes; it is much easier to grasp a large handle than a small one. An electric toothbrush can save some effort. If reach is a problem, mount long handles on combs and brushes. You can build up nail clippers with long wooden handles to make them easier to use. If you mount a nail brush on suction cups, it will stay put while you scrub. An electric razor is often more manageable than a hand one, and razor holders to improve your grip are available from major manufacturers such as Remington, Sunbeam, and Norelco.

When to See the Health Professional for Problems with Bathing and Hygiene

- *After home treatment, you still need assistance from someone else in order to bathe and clean up.*
- *After home treatment, the problem is still getting worse.*

Many women prefer a cream-type depilatory for their legs. There are even Velcro hair curlers that can be worked with one hand.

You won't need to make use of all these tricks, of course, but they are included to give you an idea of the many ways in which you can simplify an essential everyday activity.

WHAT TO EXPECT FROM THE HEALTH PROFESSIONAL

The occupational therapist can suggest additional ideas and will know where to obtain needed gadgets. The social worker can sometimes help in obtaining funds or in finding used equipment. Remember that devices required for your disability can be tax deductible, which decreases the cost to you. These expenditures are worth the cost.

40/ *Turning Handles and Opening Doors*

With disability, the world can sometimes seem like an unfriendly place. Products designed for style rather than for function make many activities difficult even if you have a good thumb and a strong grip, and if you don't, you're in trouble. Some of these design features are totally unnecessary; before you buy, check products for good functional design. The key words are "safe," "sturdy," "efficient," "easy to work," "easy to fix." Look for these features when you buy a house, a motor home, a car, shoes, a toothbrush, or anything else. As a consumer, you speak with your dollars, and that is the language the designers ultimately listen to. When you run into something particularly outrageous, write the manufacturer. Write a consumer group. Write a government consumer agency. Keep the pressure on.

Meanwhile, here are a few hints to help you with the world as it now is.

HOME TREATMENT

The old car door push button is truly a beast. You have to push with a thumb and pull with the hand at the same time, and the thumb action is against a hard spring. Sometimes you will be able to push the button with your palm. If not, try both thumbs at once. Or you can have a handyperson make an aluminum gripper that hooks on the door handle and lets you lever the push button in. New car door handles are much easier than those of older cars; if you have trouble with the catch, a T-shaped piece of wood will let you pry it out.

A handle with pointed bars, like some shower handles, can also be worked with a lever—a bamboo or aluminum tube works well. When you buy new fixtures, however, get ones with a single lever that controls both water force and temperature. Remember the lever, because it is the answer to many frustrating problems.

Learn to use the palm when you grip. If you press on a handle, you get a surprising amount of friction. By then rotating the whole hand, you can turn the handle without actually gripping it. You can use a little grip too, but let the friction of the hand do most of the work.

Keys can be built up with an added wood handle to make them easier to turn. But don't forget the graphite. With a little lock oil or graphite in the lock, the whole job becomes much easier.

When to See the Health Professional for Problems with Grip

■ *After home treatment, you still need assistance from someone else in order to turn handles or open doors.*

■ *After home treatment, the problem is still there and getting worse.*

WHAT TO EXPECT FROM THE HEALTH PROFESSIONAL

The occupational therapist can give you additional adaptive suggestions and is a good person to ask about where to obtain some of the materials you need.

41/ *Opening Jars*

Some people think that applesauce jars are the worst. Others give the award to catsup bottles. Then there are the can openers, and the plastic or cellophane wrappers that won't tear. These are problems for everyone. Domestic battles rage over the opening of a difficult jar on a difficult day. And if your grip strength is decreased because of arthritis or other disability, you may need some tricks to help you out (with the jars, not the domestic battles).

Don't minimize this problem because it seems so ordinary and so unimportant. Frustration at a trivial task is more marked than with a larger one. Your feeling of helplessness before a stubborn jar is not good for you. So learn the tricks.

HOME TREATMENT

Mount a wedge-shaped gripper on the kitchen wall; this allows you to turn the jar easily with two hands while the lid is securely held. Break the suction on vacuum lids, such as applesauce, with a "lid lifter" available in houseware departments everywhere. You can use the blunt end of a "church key" beer can opener. Use a fork handle as a lever to pull up ring-top openers.

For boxes, lay the box on its side and cut the top off with a knife. Keep several set of scissors around, and use them for sealed plastic or cellophane. Get an electric can opener; the ones that have a power stroke to pierce the can will save additional effort. If you use a hand can opener, make sure that the handles are large and easy to grip.

Practice opening jars with your palm. The friction between lid and palm enables you to get more force than you can with just the grip. You can use a little grip to assist the palm friction. This simple but unfamiliar action can make opening jars a lot easier.

When to See the Health Professional for Problems with Jars

- *After home treatment, you still need assistance from someone else in order to open moderately difficult cans or jars.*
- *After home treatment, the problem is still there and getting worse.*

WHAT TO EXPECT FROM THE HEALTH PROFESSIONAL

The occupational therapist can suggest some additional tricks and is a good person to ask about where to obtain items in your area. Everything you need to conquer this particular problem is probably available at a nearby store, so the health professional will not be of as much assistance with this problem as well as with some others. You have to learn to look for items with care, anticipating how well they will work with your particular disability.

42/ *Eating*

Eating problems pose a most fundamental frustration. Eating is a complicated task that involves mental activity, physical abilities, and body reflexes to carry the food to and through the stomach. Interruption of the sequence at any point can cause a problem. The difficulty for the person with arthritis or disability may involve cutting the food, getting the food to the mouth, chewing, or swallowing. These can be serious problems. Eating is a social occasion as well as a biological necessity, and eating gracefully without self-consciousness is a social skill we take for granted.

HOME TREATMENT

The suggestions here are just to get you started. As with other daily activities, your own solutions will require a bit of personalizing and ingenuity. There are several ways to make it easier to cut your food. Attractive utensils are available with big handles that enable you to get a better grip. If the plate is placed on a damp sponge cloth or a thin disc of rubber, it will not slip while you are cutting; this may give you an extra hand for the knife as well as a feeling of greater security. Don't forget that a sharp knife will cut more easily than a dull one (but be careful). Foods can be selected that are equally good in taste but easier to cut. High-friction plastic placed between the plate and the table can also help keep the plate steady while you cut. These measures can help at stirring or opening as well as in cutting.

In getting food to the mouth, built-up utensil handles are again useful. *T*-handled cups make for an easier grip, as does a terry cloth coaster around a glass. Long-handled utensils are needed by some, while angled utensils are easier for others. A swivel spoon can be used by people unable to twist their wrist to bring liquid to the mouth. Straws are sometimes an easy way to drink, and an ordinary pencil pocket clip can help you attach the straw to the side of the glass to make it even simpler.

Chewing problems can arise from arthritis of the jaw joints or from problems with the teeth or the chewing muscles. Good dental care is essential. Selection of food that can be chewed easily is one way to avoid the problem.

Swallowing can be affected in several ways. In myositis, the upper swallowing muscles may not work. In scleroderma, the muscles in the lower gullet may not pass a smooth swallowing wave. Medicines may irritate the stomach and not let food leave the stomach efficiently. Chew carefully and slowly and swallow carefully. If the problem seems to be low in the gullet, an antacid may be helpful. Take small, frequent meals, use softer textured foods, take liquids with meals, and eat and chew slowly. Try not eating for the two or three hours before bedtime if you have pain behind the breast bone when you eat. Having pain when you eat is an indication that you should see the doctor, as is any weight loss due to difficulty in eating.

When to See the Health Professional for Problems with Eating

- *You have had weight loss of over five pounds.*
- *You have significant pain when eating.*
- *Despite home treatment, you still need someone to assist you in order to eat.*

WHAT TO EXPECT FROM THE HEALTH PROFESSIONAL

The occupational therapist is knowledgeable about adaptive aids and where to get them. The social worker may be needed in severe cases to locate public resources. The doctor is necessary if chewing or swallowing problems are causing major difficulty. X-rays of the jaw and the temporal mandibular joint may be taken. An upper GI series is an x-ray of the esophagus, stomach, and duodenum, and it may help identify a problem in these areas.

43/ *Managing Stairs*

In some living environments there are no stairs. This is true of the single-level house or homes equipped with elevators. In other situations, the ability to climb stairs is essential to independent life. Stairs sometimes must be used several times a day; even the bathroom, if upstairs, can require this activity. Problems with the knees, with the hips, or with the quadriceps muscles in the thigh are usually responsible for difficulty with stairs. Thus loss of ability to climb stairs is a signal for increased attention to your exercise program and to your medical care; a minor problem has just become major.

HOME TREATMENT

Often your first approach should be to check your medication program with your doctor. Are you taking needed medication regularly? Does your doctor have further suggestions? Are you working on your quadriceps-strengthening exercises? Might a steroid injection of an inflamed knee be of benefit? Is this the signal to seriously consider a surgical procedure on that bad hip or knee?

Sometimes you can rearrange your environment quite a bit. Should you move? An apartment with an elevator? A ranch-style house with a single level? Should you remodel? A downstairs bedroom and bath? A ramp in the garden, gently graded? Such changes, while perhaps expensive, can sometimes render use of stairs unnecessary.

Can you improve your stairs? Be sure that you have a rail or banister on each side so that you can steady yourself and push a bit with your arms. Sometimes installation of a center rail will help you by allowing you to use both hands at once.

The split-riser trick also helps some people. If your problem is that the steps are just too high, you can have a carpenter install split risers so that half of each step is raised half a step, alternating left and right. Then you can climb the stairs, moving back and forth, without ever having to go up a full step at a time.

The rules for climbing stairs if you are having trouble: one at a time, with both feet on the same stair before trying the next one. Go up with the best leg first; go down with the best leg first. Use the same techniques for curbs.

Another possibility is installation of a home elevator or a lift that goes up on a banister. These are quite expensive and are thus out of reach for all but a few. For these few, remember that the cost may be tax-deductible if recommended by your doctor. If you are considering one of these expensive changes, you should think again through the options of moving or remodeling.

When to See the Health Professional for Problems with Stairs

- *Despite home treatment, you require assistance from another person for necessary stair-climbing activities.*
- *Despite home treatment, the problem is still there and getting worse.*

WHAT TO EXPECT FROM THE HEALTH PROFESSIONAL

The occupational therapist may have some additional suggestions for you and will know where to obtain materials. The social worker may be able to help with sources of financing. Your doctor may refer you to a specialist such as a rheumatologist (doctor who specializes in care of the joints) or an orthopedic surgeon (surgeon who performs surgery on the joints) for additional suggestions or procedures.

44/ *Difficulty Walking*

Walking is central to almost every other activity. Thus the ability to walk *must* be preserved. If walking is impaired, the muscles become weak, the bones lose calcium, the legs tend to swell, friends are more distant, and the easiest tasks become formidable. This cycle can further reduce your health and increase your dependency on others. So if you are having trouble walking and you can't take care of the problem yourself, have a long talk with your doctor. Usually something can be done. The longer that you have been unable to walk, the more difficult the solution.

With some kinds of arthritis, fatigue can cause a decrease in your desire to walk; you must fight against this. Or problems with the ball of the foot, the ankles, the knees, the hips, or the walking muscles can be responsible for the difficulty. Problems with walking are sometimes a medical problem and sometimes partly a social one.

HOME TREATMENT

Be sure that the treatment for your arthritis or other disability is right. Are you taking your medicine regularly? Do you need a change in medication? Could problems be a side effect of a medication? Is your exercise program being pursued diligently? Is a single joint causing the trouble? Could this joint be injected with cortisone? Do you perhaps have a joint infection? Is this the time to consider surgery for that bad knee or bad hip? These and similar questions can help you decide on a strategy to get walking again.

A cane is the simplest aid to walking. It is usually held in the hand opposite an affected hip and on the most comfortable side for a bad knee. The usual C-handled cane is not really designed to be held easily, so you might prefer one with a functional grip handle. Some handles may need to be built up with tape to allow good grip.

Crutches give somewhat more support but are more cumbersome. When using crutches, your weight should not be on your armpits but on your arms. The armpit is laced with fragile nerves and blood vessels, and pressure there for very long can cause damage. You may have to pad the grip or fit a knob to the crutch to get a good grip. If your grip is not too good, forearm platform crutches can help you take the weight on the forearm. Bags can be attached to the crutch to allow small items to be carried—you just don't have enough hands for a purse or package otherwise.

Walkers give stable support but are difficult to use for long distances. They are most useful about the house or while you are getting back on your feet after a flare up or after an operation.

Don't forget about the importance of correct footwear. If foot pain is limiting your walking, you will want to refer to some of the hints given in Problems 10, 11, and 12. Hip problems are discussed in Problem 8, knee problems in Problem 9, and ankle problems in Problem 10.

When to See the Doctor for Difficulty in Walking

- *Despite home treatment, you are unable to do activities that you would like to do because of difficulty in walking.*
- *You are unable to walk as much as you would like because of pain.*

Then there are gliders and wheel chairs; we recommend that you talk with your physical therapist or occupational therapist for specific techniques for using these.

Review the particular parts of your exercise program. If your knees won't straighten entirely, they need to be systematically stretched many times each day to try and recover that lost range of motion. Walking itself, even short distances, is the best exercise for your walking muscles. Force yourself twice a day to walk to the point where you have some discomfort, of course being very careful not to fall. The stronger your body, the better you will be able to handle this problem.

WHAT TO EXPECT FROM THE HEALTH PROFESSIONAL

The physical therapist will help you get started with appliances for walking assistance and can instruct you in exercises to strengthen your legs. The occupational therapist can help with additional adaptive devices. Social workers may assist in mobilizing community resources to help you. Your doctor will want to take a very serious look at your treatment program to ensure that all the right things are being done. Remember, whatever your age, if a specific bad joint or even two or three joints are the root of the problem, there are now good surgical procedures that can help.

45/ *Difficulty Sleeping*

Good sleep is an important part of good health. Too little sleep is bad; too much sleep is bad also. Even more important is getting the right kind of sleep.

We need less sleep as we grow older. The eight hours a day that are appropriate for the young adult decrease to seven in our 60s and to six or less in our 70s and beyond. Of course, individual requirements vary greatly, but practically no one should need more than eight hours at any age.

There are different kinds of sleep. During light sleep stages we are nearly awake. We dream, and our eyes move from side to side as though watching the action. This is called rapid-eye-movement (or REM) sleep. In the deepest stages we lie motionless, in "sleep paralysis." During the night we constantly move back and forth between the stages, with more deep sleep periods early in the night and more light sleep periods toward morning. The key to restful, restorative sleep is to get enough periods of deep sleep.

HOME TREATMENT

Physical exercise is the most important promoter of good deep sleep. Our bodies are designed to be used, then rested, then used again. You need to be physically tired at the end of the day to sleep well. Work the activities and exercise progressions described in Chapter 7.

Caffeine is a big offender, even though everybody knows about it. Remember that as you grow older all drugs last longer in your body. Caffeine can still be in your bloodstream after six hours. Watch out for caffeine in coffee (of course), tea, colas and other soft drinks, chocolate (often neglected), and in over-the-counter pain medications.

Other drugs also are frequent offenders. Allergy medicines and cold medicines often contain stimulants like ephedrine or metanephrine that can keep you awake. The effects of these stimulants can last several days in some people. Almost any prescription drugs (and many non-prescription drugs) can cause insomnia in some people. Suspect everything.

"Paradoxical" reactions occur in older individuals with some frequency. With these reactions, a medicine given to help you sleep actually keeps you awake. Tranquilizers and sleeping pills are notorious for causing such paradoxical reactions in senior patients.

In general sleeping pills are *not* a good way to help you sleep better. Often they cause you to not get the right kind of sleep or prevent your sleeping from cycling normally between the different stages of sleep.

If a medical problem is keeping you awake by causing discomfort, you need to pay attention to treating the medical problem first. Arthritis, Parkinson's disease, leg pains, and hiatal hernias are some medical conditions that can cause sleep problems. Check out the appropriate sections in this book, and if that doesn't work see the doctor.

When to See the Doctor for Difficulty Sleeping

- *Your sleep disturbance is associated with feelings of worthlessness and depression.*
- *Despite a full program of home treatment you are still having a major problem with insomnia.*

Remember your sleeping environment; you want it quiet and comfortable. Keep clutter, work, and other reminders of the stressful day away. Sometimes music played very low can help. Read for a while with the bedside light. Practice relaxation techniques. Develop for yourself the routines that work best.

If you are having feelings of worthlessness and depression, whether or not you have been thinking of suicide, see the doctor. Depression is common and usually interferes with sleep. Typically the depressed person can go to sleep normally but wakes up in the middle of the night and has trouble getting back to sleep. Often during these waking periods a single thought keeps going around and around in your head, and you can't think of anything else. There is a good treatment for depression, from exercise to drugs, but you should talk the problem over with your doctor.

WHAT TO EXPECT AT THE DOCTOR'S OFFICE

Considerations such as those given in the "Home Treatment" section will be discussed and suggestions made. The conscientious doctor will prescribe sleeping pills only as a last resort—they can make you drowsy during the day, have side effects, and sometimes interact with other drugs. If depression is present, antidepressant medications may be prescribed. For patients with particularly severe problems, there are now doctors who specialize in sleep disorders and sleep clinics; these doctors have sophisticated approaches and a variety of new treatments that help many patients.

PART IV

Appendixes

Forms for Advance Directives

Some Surprising Statistics

For Further Reading

Forms for Advance Directives

My Living Will and Directive to My Physician

Springing Durable Power of Attorney for Health Care (Not Valid in California)

Springing Durable Power of Attorney (Health Care) (California)

Springing Durable Power of Attorney for Financial/Asset Management

1/ Living Will

My Living Will and Directive to My Physicians

Directive made this ________ day of ______________, 19____.

I, ____,
(name)

residing in the County of ______________________________,

State of ____,

being of sound mind, willfully and voluntarily make known my desire that my life shall not be artificially prolonged under the circumstances set forth below and do hereby declare:

1. If at any time I should have an incurable injury, disease, or illness certified to be a terminal condition by two physicians, and where the application of life-sustaining procedures would serve only to artificially prolong the moment of my death and where my physician determines that my death is imminent whether or not life-sustaining procedures are utilized, I direct that such procedures be withheld or withdrawn, and that I be permitted to die naturally.

2. In the absence of my ability to give directions regarding the use of such life-sustaining procedures, it is my intention that this directive shall be honored by my family and physician(s) as the final expression of my legal right to refuse medical or surgical treatment and accept the consequences from such refusal.

3. I have been diagnosed and notified at least 14 days ago as having a terminal condition by ______________________, M.D.,
(physician's name)

whose address is ____
(address)

____,

and whose telephone number is ______________________.

I understand that if I have not filled in the physician's name and address, it shall be presumed that I did not have a terminal condition when I made out this directive.

(continued on following page)

4. I understand the full import of this directive and I am emotionally and mentally competent to make this directive.

Dated: ______________________________, 19____

____
PRINCIPAL **(signature)**

____
(city, county, and state of residence)

WITNESSES

This declarant has been personally known to me and I believe him/her to be of sound mind.

____
WITNESS 1

Residing at ______________________________

____

____
WITNESS 2

Residing at ______________________________

____

2/ Power of Attorney for Health Care

Springing Durable Power of Attorney for Health Care (Not Valid in California)

1. CREATION OF DURABLE POWER OF ATTORNEY

To my family, relatives, friends and my physicians, health care providers, community care facilities and any other person who may have an interest or duty in my medical care or treatment:

I, ____,
(name)

being of sound mind, willfully and voluntarily intend to create by this document a durable power of attorney for my health care by appointing the person designated as my attorney-in-fact to make health care decisions for me in the event I become incapacitated and am unable to make health care decisions for myself. This power of attorney shall not be affected by my subsequent incapacity.

2. DESIGNATION OF ATTORNEY-IN-FACT

The person designated to be my attorney-in-fact for health care in the event I become incapacitated

is ____
(name)

of ____.
(address)

If ____________________ for any reason shall fail to serve or ceases to serve as my attorney-in-fact for health care,

____ of
(name)

____
(address)

shall be my attorney-in-fact for health care.

3. EFFECTIVE ON INCAPACITY

This durable power of attorney shall become effective in the event I become incapacitated and am unable to make health care decisions for myself, in which case it shall be-

(continued on following page)

come effective as of the date of the written statement by a physician, as provided in paragraph 4.

4. DETERMINATION OF INCAPACITY

(a) The determination that I have become incapacitated and am unable to make health care decisions shall be made in writing by a licensed physician. If possible, the determination shall be made

by ________________, ______________________________.
(name) (address)

(b) In the event that a licensed physician has made a written determination that I have become incapacitated and am not able to make health care decisions for myself, that written statement shall be attached to the original document of this durable power of attorney.

5. AUTHORITY OF MY ATTORNEY-IN-FACT

My attorney-in-fact shall have all lawful authority permissible to make health care decisions for me, including the authority to consent, or withdraw consent or refuse consent to any care, treatment, service or procedure to maintain, diagnose or treat my physical or mental condition,

EXCEPT ____

____

____

6. INSPECTION AND DISCLOSURE INFORMATION OF RELATING MY PHYSICAL OR MENTAL HEALTH

Subject to any limitations in this document, my attorney-in-fact has the power and authority to do all of the following:

(a) Request, review, and receive any information, verbal or written, regarding my physical or mental health, including, but not limited to, medical and hospital records.

(b) Execute on my behalf any releases or other documents that may be required in order to obtain this information.

(c) Consent to the disclosure of this information.

7. SIGNING DOCUMENTS, WAIVERS, AND RELEASES

Where necessary to implement health care decisions that my attorney-in-fact is authorized by this document to make, my attorney-in-fact has the power and authority to execute on my behalf all of the following:

(a) Documents titled or purporting to be a "Refusal to Permit Treatment" and "Leaving Hospital Against Medical Advice."

(b) Any necessary waiver or release from liability required by a hospital or physician.

8. DURATION

I intend that this Durable Power of Attorney remain effective until my death, or until revoked by me in writing.

Executed this ________ day of ____________________, 19____

at ____.

____

PRINCIPAL

WITNESSES

I declare that the principal is personally known to me, that the principal signed or acknowledged this durable power of attorney in my presence, that the principal appears to be of sound mind and under no duress, fraud, or undue influence.

I further declare that I am not related to the principal by blood, marriage, or adoption, and to the best of my knowledge, I am not entitled to any part of the estate of that prin-

(continued on following page)

cipal upon the death of the principal under a Will now existing or by operation of law.

____________________________ of ________________________
WITNESS 1
____

____________________________ of ________________________
WITNESS 2
____

NOTARIZATION

State of ____

County of ____

On this ________ day of _____________ in the year 19____,

before me a Notary Public, State of ______________________,

duly commissioned and sworn, personally appeared

______________________________________, personally known

to me (or proved to me on the basis of satisfactory evidence) to be the person whose name is subscribed to in the within instrument, and acknowledged to me that

_____________________________________ executed the same.

IN WITNESS WHEREOF, I have hereunto set my hand and affixed my official seal

in the ____________________ County of ____________________.

on the date set forth above in this certificate.

____
NOTARY PUBLIC
State of ____

My commission expires ____________________________________

3/ Power of Attorney for Health Care (California)

Springing Durable Power of Attorney for Health Care (CALIFORNIA)

WARNING TO PERSON EXECUTING THIS DOCUMENT

THIS IS AN IMPORTANT LEGAL DOCUMENT. IT CREATES A DURABLE POWER OF ATTORNEY FOR HEALTH CARE. BEFORE EXECUTING THIS DOCUMENT, YOU SHOULD KNOW THESE IMPORTANT FACTS.

THIS DOCUMENT GIVES THE PERSON YOU DESIGNATE AS YOUR AGENT (THE ATTORNEY-IN-FACT) THE POWER TO MAKE HEALTH CARE DECISIONS FOR YOU. YOUR AGENT MUST ACT CONSISTENTLY WITH YOUR DESIRES AS STATED IN THIS DOCUMENT OR OTHERWISE MADE KNOWN.

EXCEPT AS YOU OTHERWISE SPECIFY IN THIS DOCUMENT, THIS DOCUMENT GIVES YOUR AGENT THE POWER TO CONSENT TO YOUR DOCTOR NOT GIVING TREATMENT OR STOPPING TREATMENT NECESSARY TO KEEP YOU ALIVE.

NOTWITHSTANDING THIS DOCUMENT, YOU HAVE THE RIGHT TO MAKE MEDICAL AND OTHER HEALTH CARE DECISIONS FOR YOURSELF SO LONG AS YOU CAN GIVE INFORMED CONSENT WITH RESPECT TO THE PARTICULAR DECISION. IN ADDITION, NO TREATMENT MAY BE GIVEN TO YOU OVER YOUR OBJECTION, AND HEALTH CARE NECESSARY TO KEEP YOU ALIVE MAY NOT BE STOPPED OR WITHHELD IF YOU OBJECT AT THIS TIME.

THIS DOCUMENT GIVES YOUR AGENT AUTHORITY TO CONSENT, TO REFUSE TO CONSENT, OR TO WITHDRAW CONSENT TO ANY CARE, TREATMENT, SERVICE, OR PROCEDURE TO MAINTAIN, DIAGNOSE, OR TREAT A PHYSICAL OR MENTAL CONDITION. THIS POWER IS SUBJECT TO ANY STATEMENT OF YOUR DESIRES AND ANY LIMITATIONS THAT YOU INCLUDE IN THIS DOCUMENT. YOU MAY STATE IN THIS DOCUMENT ANY TYPES OF TREATMENT THAT YOU DO NOT DESIRE. IN ADDITION, A COURT CAN TAKE AWAY THE POWER OF YOUR AGENT TO MAKE HEALTH CARE DECISIONS FOR YOU IF YOUR AGENT (1) AUTHORIZES ANYTHING THAT IS ILLEGAL, (2) ACTS CONTRARY TO YOUR KNOWN DESIRES, OR (3) WHERE YOUR DESIRES ARE NOT KNOWN, DOES ANYTHING THAT IS CLEARLY CONTRARY TO YOUR BEST INTERESTS.

UNLESS YOU SPECIFY A SHORTER PERIOD IN THIS DOCUMENT, THIS POWER WILL EXIST FOR SEVEN YEARS FROM THE DATE YOU

EXECUTE THIS DOCUMENT AND, IF YOU ARE UNABLE TO MAKE HEALTH CARE DECISIONS FOR YOURSELF AT THE TIME WHEN THIS SEVEN-YEAR PERIOD ENDS, THIS POWER WILL CONTINUE TO EXIST UNTIL THE TIME WHEN YOU BECOME ABLE TO MAKE HEALTH CARE DECISIONS FOR YOURSELF.

YOU HAVE THE RIGHT TO REVOKE THE AUTHORITY OF YOUR AGENT BY NOTIFYING YOUR AGENT OR YOUR TREATING DOCTOR, HOSPITAL, OR OTHER HEALTH CARE PROVIDER ORALLY OR IN WRITING OF THE REVOCATION.

YOUR AGENT HAS THE RIGHT TO EXAMINE YOUR MEDICAL RECORDS AND TO CONSENT TO THEIR DISCLOSURE UNLESS YOU LIMIT THIS RIGHT IN THIS DOCUMENT.

UNLESS YOU OTHERWISE SPECIFY IN THIS DOCUMENT, THIS DOCUMENT GIVES YOUR AGENT THE POWER AFTER YOU DIE TO (1) AUTHORIZE AN AUTOPSY, (2) DONATE YOUR BODY OR PARTS THEREOF FOR TRANSPLANT OR THERAPEUTIC OR EDUCATIONAL OR SCIENTIFIC PURPOSES, AND (3) DIRECT THE DISPOSITION OF YOUR REMAINS.

IF THERE IS ANYTHING IN THIS DOCUMENT THAT YOU DO NOT UNDERSTAND, YOU SHOULD ASK A LAWYER TO EXPLAIN IT TO YOU.

THIS POWER OF ATTORNEY WILL NOT BE VALID FOR MAKING HEALTH CARE DECISIONS UNLESS IT IS EITHER (1) SIGNED BY TWO QUALIFIED ADULT WITNESSES WHO PERSONALLY KNOW YOU AND WHO ARE PRESENT WHEN YOU SIGN OR ACKNOWLEDGE YOUR SIGNATURE OR (2) ACKNOWLEDGED BEFORE A NOTARY PUBLIC IN CALIFORNIA.

DURABLE POWER OF ATTORNEY FOR HEALTH CARE

1. CREATION OF DURABLE POWER OF ATTORNEY

To my family, relatives, friends and my physicians, health care providers, community care facilities and any other person who may have an interest or duty in my medical care or treatment:

I, ____
(name)

being of sound mind, willfully and voluntarily intend to

create by this document a durable power of attorney for my health care by appointing the person designated as my attorney-in-fact to make health care decisions for me in the event I become incapacitated and am unable to make health care decisions for myself. This power of attorney shall not be affected by my subsequent incapacity.

2. DESIGNATION OF ATTORNEY-IN-FACT

The person designated to be my attorney-in-fact for health care in the event I become incapacitated

is ____

of ____.
(address)

If ______________________________________ for any reason
(name)

shall fail to serve or ceases to serve as my attorney-in-fact

for health care, ________________________________
(name)

of ____
(address)

shall be my attorney-in-fact for health care.

3. EFFECTIVE ON INCAPACITY

This durable power of attorney shall become effective in the event I become incapacitated and am unable to make health care decisions for myself, in which case it shall become effective as of the date of the written statement by a physician, as provided in Paragraph 4.

4. DETERMINATION OF INCAPACITY

The determination that I have become incapacitated and am unable to make health care decisions shall be made in writing by a licensed physician. If possible, the determination shall be made by

____
(name of physician)

____.
(address)

5. AUTHORITY OF MY ATTORNEY-IN-FACT

My attorney-in-fact shall have all lawful authority permissible to make health care decisions for me, including the authority to consent, or withdraw consent or refuse consent to any care, treatment, service or procedure to maintain, diagnose or treat my physical or mental condition,

EXCEPT ____

____

____

6. INSPECTION AND DISCLOSURE OF INFORMATION RELATING TO MY PHYSICAL OR MENTAL HEALTH

Subject to any limitations in this document, my attorney-in-fact has the power and authority to do all of the following:

(a) Request, review, and receive any information, verbal or written, regarding my physical or mental health, including, but not limited to, medical and hospital records.

(b) Execute on my behalf any releases or other documents that may be required in order to obtain this information.

(c) Consent to the disclosure of this information.

7. SIGNING DOCUMENTS, WAIVERS, AND RELEASES

Where necessary to implement the health care decisions that my attorney-in-fact is authorized by this document to make, my attorney-in-fact has the power and authority to execute on my behalf all of the following:

(a) Documents titled or purporting to be a "Refusal to Permit Treatment" and "Leaving Hospital Against Medical Advice."

(b) Any necessary waiver or release from liability required by a hospital or physician.

8. DURATION

I intend that this Durable Power of Attorney remain effective until my death, or until revoked by me in writing.

Executed this ________ day of ________________. 19____

at ____.

____
PRINCIPAL

STATEMENT OF WITNESSES

(READ CAREFULLY BEFORE SIGNING. You can sign as a witness only if you personally know the principal or the identity of the principal is proved to you by convincing evidence.)

(To have convincing evidence of the identity of the principal, you must be presented with and reasonably rely on any one or more of the following:

(1) An identification card or driver's license issued by the California Department of Motor Vehicles that is current or has been issued within five years.

(2) A passport issued by the Department of State of the United States that is current or has been issued within five years.

(3) Any of the following documents if the document is current or has been issued within five years and contains a photograph and description of the person named on it, is signed by the person, and bears a serial or other identifying number:

(a) A passport issued by a foreign government that has been stamped by the United States Immigration and Naturalization Service.

(b) A driver's license issued by a state other than California or by a Canadian or Mexican public agency authorized to issue drivers' licenses.

(c) An identification card issued by a state other than California.

(d) An identification cared issued by any branch of the armed forces of the United States.

(Other kinds of proof of identity are not allowed.)

I declare under penalty of perjury under the laws of California that the person who signed or acknowledged this document is personally known to me (or proved to me on the basis of convincing evidence) to be the principal, that the principal signed or acknowledged this Durable Power of Attorney in my presence, that the principal appears to be of sound mind and under no duress, fraud, or undue influence, that I am not the person appointed as attorney-in-fact by this document, and that I am not a health care provider, an employee of health care provider, the operator of a community care facility, nor an employee of an operator of a community care facility.

I further declare under penalty of perjury under the laws of California that I am not related to the principal by blood, marriage, or adoption, and to the best of my knowledge, I am not entitled to any part of the estate of the principal upon the death of the principal under a will now existing or by operation of law.

Signature: ______________________________

Print Name: ______________________________

Residence Address: ______________________________

Date: ______________________________

STATEMENT OF PATIENT ADVOCATE OR OMBUDSMAN

(If you are a patient in a skilled nursing facility, one of the witnesses must be a patient advocate or ombudsman. The following statement is required only if you are a patient in a skilled nursing facility—a health care facility that provides the following basic services: Skilled nursing care and supportive care to patients whose primary need is for availability of skilled nursing care on an extended basis. The patient advocate or ombudsman must sign both parts of the "Statement of Witnesses" above and must also sign the following statement.)

I further declare under penalty of perjury under the laws of California that I am a patient advocate or ombudsman as designated by the State Department of Aging and that I am serving as a witness as required by subdivision (f) of Section 2432 of the Civil Code.

Signature: ______________________________

[or the durable power of attorney for health care is notarized with the following form:]

State of ______________________________)

______________________________) ss

County of ______________________________)

On this ________ day of ______________, in the year 19_____,

before me, ______________________________, personally appeared
(name of notary public)

______________________________, personally known to me
(name of principal)

(or proved to me on the basis of satisfactory evidence) to be the person whose name is subscribed to this instrument,

and acknowledged that ______________ executed it. I declare
(he/she)

under penalty of perjury that the person whose name is subscribed to this instrument appears to be of sound mind and under no duress, fraud, or undue influence.

____
(signature of notary public)

[*notarial seal*] Notary Public for The State of ______________

My commission expires: ______________________, 19_____.

4/ Power of Attorney for Financial Management

Springing Durable Power of Attorney for Financial/Asset Management

Recording requested by and when recorded mail to

____

____

____

WARNING TO PERSON EXECUTING THIS DOCUMENT

THIS IS AN IMPORTANT LEGAL DOCUMENT. IT CREATES A DURABLE POWER OF ATTORNEY. BEFORE EXECUTING THIS DOCUMENT, YOU SHOULD KNOW THESE IMPORTANT FACTS:

1. THIS DOCUMENT MAY PROVIDE THE PERSON YOU DESIGNATE AS YOUR ATTORNEY-IN-FACT WITH BROAD POWERS TO MANAGE, DISPOSE, SELL, AND CONVEY YOUR REAL AND PERSONAL PROPERTY AND TO BORROW MONEY USING YOUR PROPERTY AS SECURITY FOR THE LOAN.

2. THESE POWERS WILL EXIST FOR AN INDEFINITE PERIOD OF TIME UNLESS YOU LIMIT THEIR DURATION IN THIS DOCUMENT. THESE POWERS WILL CONTINUE TO EXIST NOTWITHSTANDING YOUR SUBSEQUENT DISABILITY OR INCAPACITY.

3. YOU HAVE THE RIGHT TO REVOKE OR TERMINATE THIS DURABLE POWER OF ATTORNEY.

IF THERE IS ANYTHING ABOUT THIS FORM THAT YOU DO NOT UNDERSTAND, YOU SHOULD ASK A LAWYER TO EXPLAIN IT TO YOU.

DURABLE POWER OF ATTORNEY

1. CREATION OF DURABLE POWER OF ATTORNEY

By signing this document,

I, ____,

intend to create a durable power of attorney. This durable power of attorney shall not be affected by my subsequent disability or incapacity, and shall remain effective until my death, or until revoked by me in writing.

2. EFFECTIVE DATE

This durable power of attorney shall become effective only in the event that I become incapacitated or disabled so that I am not able to manage my financial affairs in which case it shall become effective as of the date of the written statement by a physician, as provided in Paragraph 3. If the durable power of attorney becomes effective, it shall remain effective during any period when I am incapacitated or disabled until my death, or until revoked by me.

3. DETERMINATION OF INCAPACITY

The determination of whether I have become incapacitated or disabled so that I am not able to manage my financial affairs shall be made in writing by a licensed physician; if possible, the physician shall

be ____
(name)

of ____.
(address)

In the event that a licensed physician has made a written determination that I have become incapacitated or disabled and am not able to manage my own financial affairs, that written statement shall be attached to the original of this durable power of attorney.

4. DESIGNATION OF ATTORNEY-IN-FACT

If I become incapacitated or disabled so that I am not able to manage my financial affairs,

I, ____,
(name)

hereby appoint ______________________________________
(name)

of ____
(address)

as my attorney-in-fact, to act for me and in my name and for my use and benefit. Should ____________________________
(name)

for any reasons fail to serve or cease to serve as my attorney-in-fact, I appoint ______________________________________
(name)

of ____
(address)

to be my attorney-in-fact.

5. AUTHORITY OF ATTORNEY-IN-FACT

(a) Except as specified in Section 5(b), I grant my attorney-in-fact full power and authority over all my property, real and personal, and authorize ____________________
(him/her)
to do and perform all and every act which I as an owner of said property could do or perform and I hereby ratify and confirm all that my attorney-in-fact shall do or cause to be done under this durable power of attorney.

(b) My attorney-in-fact has no authority to give any of my property to, or use any of my property for the benefit of ____.
(himself/herself)

6. RELIANCE BY THIRD PARTIES

The powers conferred on my attorney-in-fact by this durable power of attorney may be exercisable by my attorney-in-fact alone, and my attorney-in-fact's signature or fact under the authority granted in this durable power of attorney may be accepted by any third person or organization as fully authorized by me and with the same force and effect as if I were personally present, competent and acting on my own behalf.

No person or organization who relies on this durable power of attorney or any representation my attorney-in-fact makes regarding ____________________ authority, including but not
(his/her)
limited to:

(i) the fact that this durable power of attorney has not been revoked;

(ii) that I, ______________________________, was competent to
(name)
execute this power of attorney;

(iii) the authority of my attorney-in-fact under this durable power of attorney:

shall incur any liability to me, my estate, heirs, successors or assigns because of such reliance on this durable power of attorney or any such representation by my attorney-in-fact.

Executed this ________ day of ________________, 19____,

at ____.

____

PRINCIPAL

WITNESSES

________________________________ of ________________

WITNESS 1

____

________________________________ of ________________

WITNESS 2

____

NOTARIZATION

State of ____

County of ______________________________________

On this ________ day of ______________ in the year 19____,

before me a Notary Public, State of ________________,
duly commissioned and sworn, personally appeared

____,

personally known to me (or proved to me on the basis of satisfactory evidence) to be the person whose name is subscribed to in the within instrument, and acknowledged to me that

______________________________ executed the same.
(he/she)

IN WITNESS WHEREOF, I have hereunto set my hand and affixed my official seal in the County of ______________ on the date set forth above in this certificate.

____

NOTARY PUBLIC

State of ______________________________

My commission expires ______________________

Some Surprising Statistics

In this book I have tried to keep complicated discussions as simple and uncluttered as possible. Everyone will not want to wade through the underlying statistics that describe aging. However, sometimes a picture, table, or chart is worth a thousand words. Following are some insights into the aging process provided in summary form. The following sixteen sets of data summarize the factual structure upon which this book has been based.

1. The Old View: Everything Declines with Age
2. Gompertz "Law": Mortality from All Causes Increases with Age
3. The Surprising Case of Pedestrian Accidents
4. Two-thirds of Deaths Are Postponable
5. The Heart Disease Epidemic That Never Came
6. The Remarkable Marathoners
7. More Lessons, This Time from Medium-Distance Runners
8. Neglected Conclusions from Scientific Studies
9. Things Are Getting Better
10. Medical Costs Don't Necessarily Rise with Age
11. Watch Out for the Last Two Months
12. Bad Habits Cost Money
13. The Compression of Morbidity—A Diagram
14. Life Expectancy for Seniors Is No Longer Rapidly Increasing
15. Will the Experts Be Wrong—Again?
16. Utilizing the Plasticity of Aging

1/ The Old View: Everything Declines with Age

For years, gerontology was described as "the science of drawing downward-sloping lines."

The reserve function *of our organs, such as heart, lungs, kidney, and nervous system, declines with age, usually at a rate of one to one-and-a-half percent per year. But, we do not often need all this reserve function in daily life. Some of this decline is due to disuse and can be improved by exercise.*

The daily function *of our organs is approximately constant throughout life. Our heart output, body acid-base balance, white blood count, breathing rates, and body chemical concentrations are maintained throughout life at about the same level.*

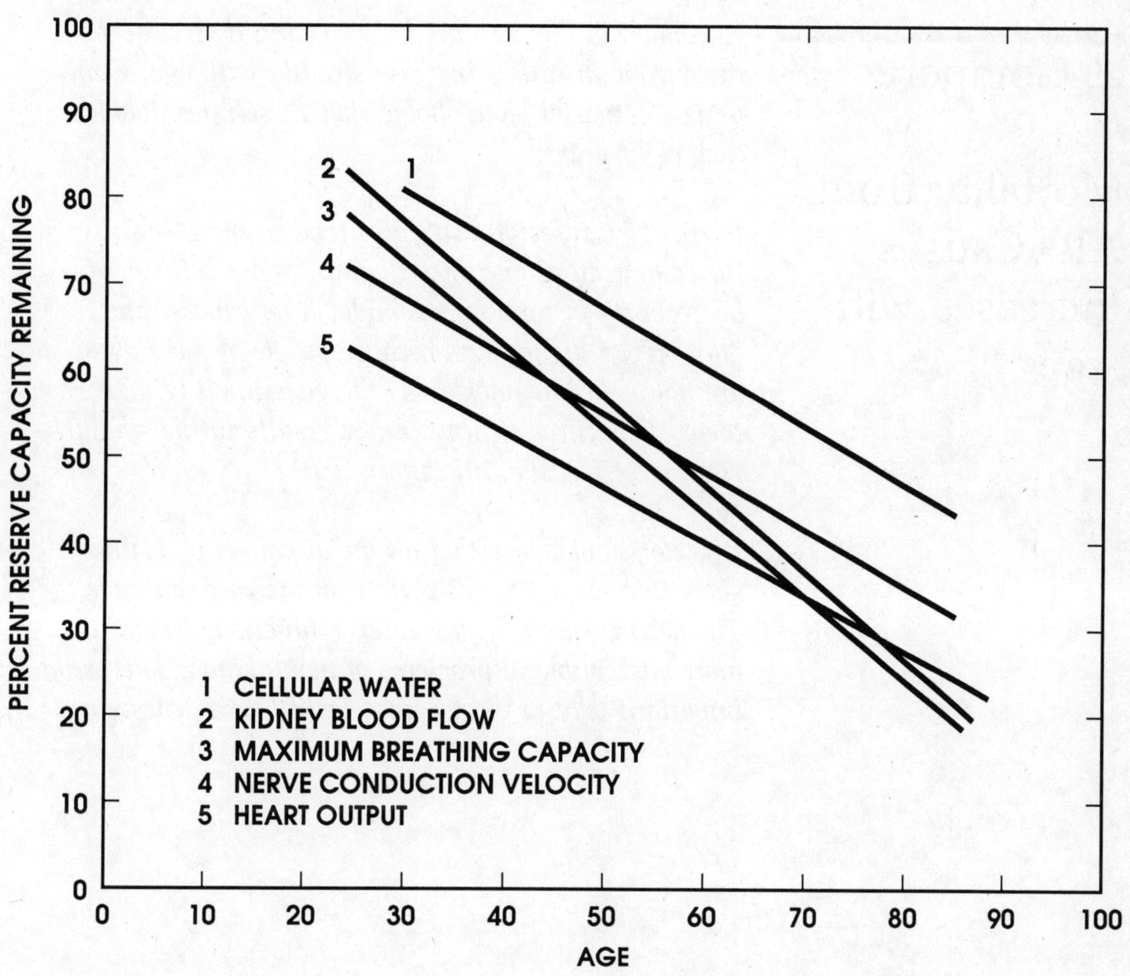

Reserve Function Slopes

2/ Gompertz "Law": Mortality from All Causes Increases with Age

As shown by the top line in the facing figure, death rates from all causes increase steadily with age. Gompertz's actuarial "law" holds that these rates double each eight years.

Particular causes of death also tend to increase in the same way. Sometimes these rates are influenced by "cohort" factors; for example, lung cancer rates "tail off" at higher ages because people of these ages are not as heavy smokers as the generation behind them. This effect of lung cancer results in the similar "tailing off" of the "all cancer" curve.

It is not coincidence that all major causes of death show this same general pattern of increase with age. The decline in our organ reserve functions leaves us more susceptible to problems of many kinds. This is one important way to view aging, frailty, and senescence.

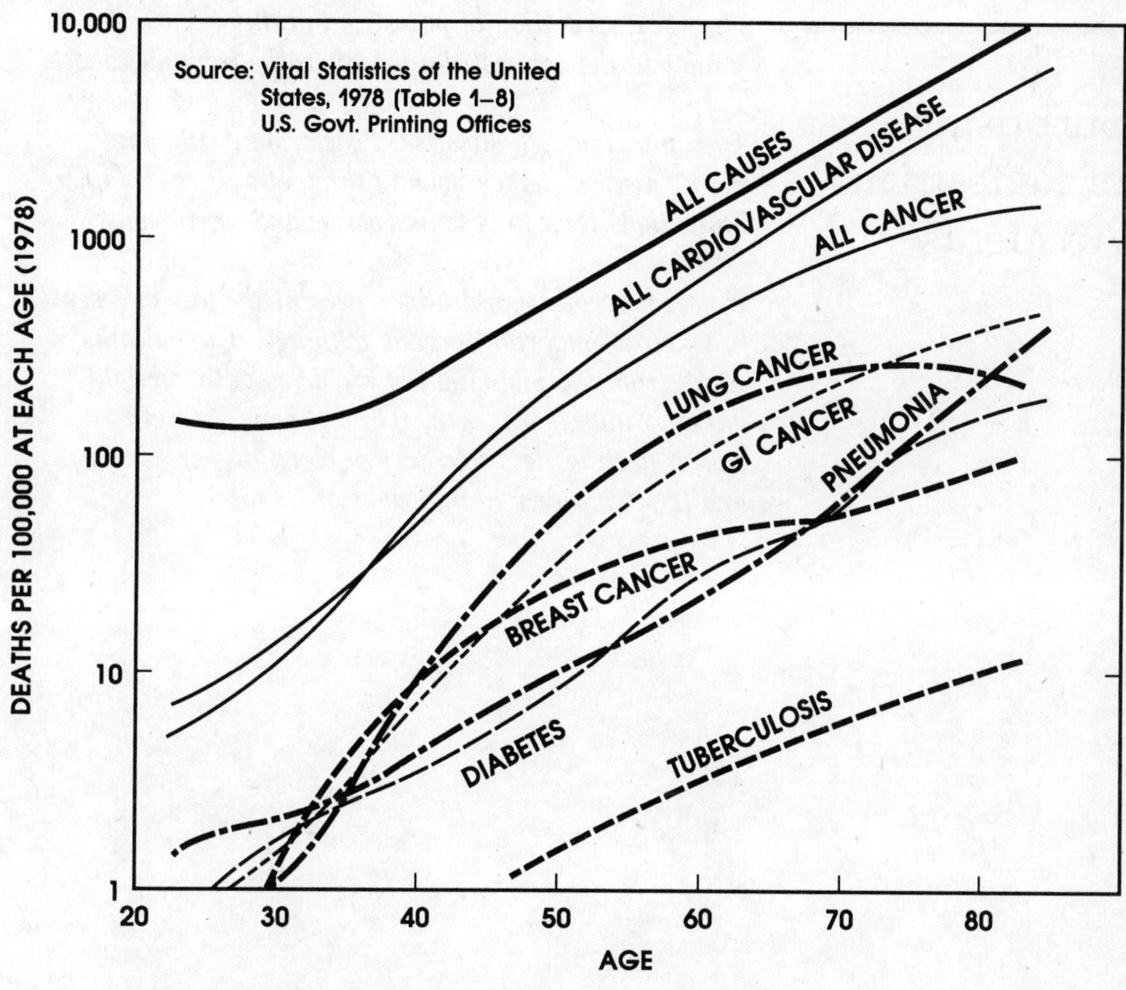

Mortality Rates by Age

3/ The Surprising Case of Pedestrian Accidents

The age distribution of pedestrian deaths is closely similar to the age distribution of deaths from all causes.

To many, this is a surprise. Pedestrian deaths are not a "disease" as we usually think of a disease. Older individuals tend to be conservative and safety-conscious.

However, pedestrian deaths represent the loss of reserve function of important organs with age. These deaths result from a combination of problems with eyesight, hearing, muscle strength, reflexes, bone strength, slower healing, less tolerance of blood loss or surgery, and less resistance to infections.

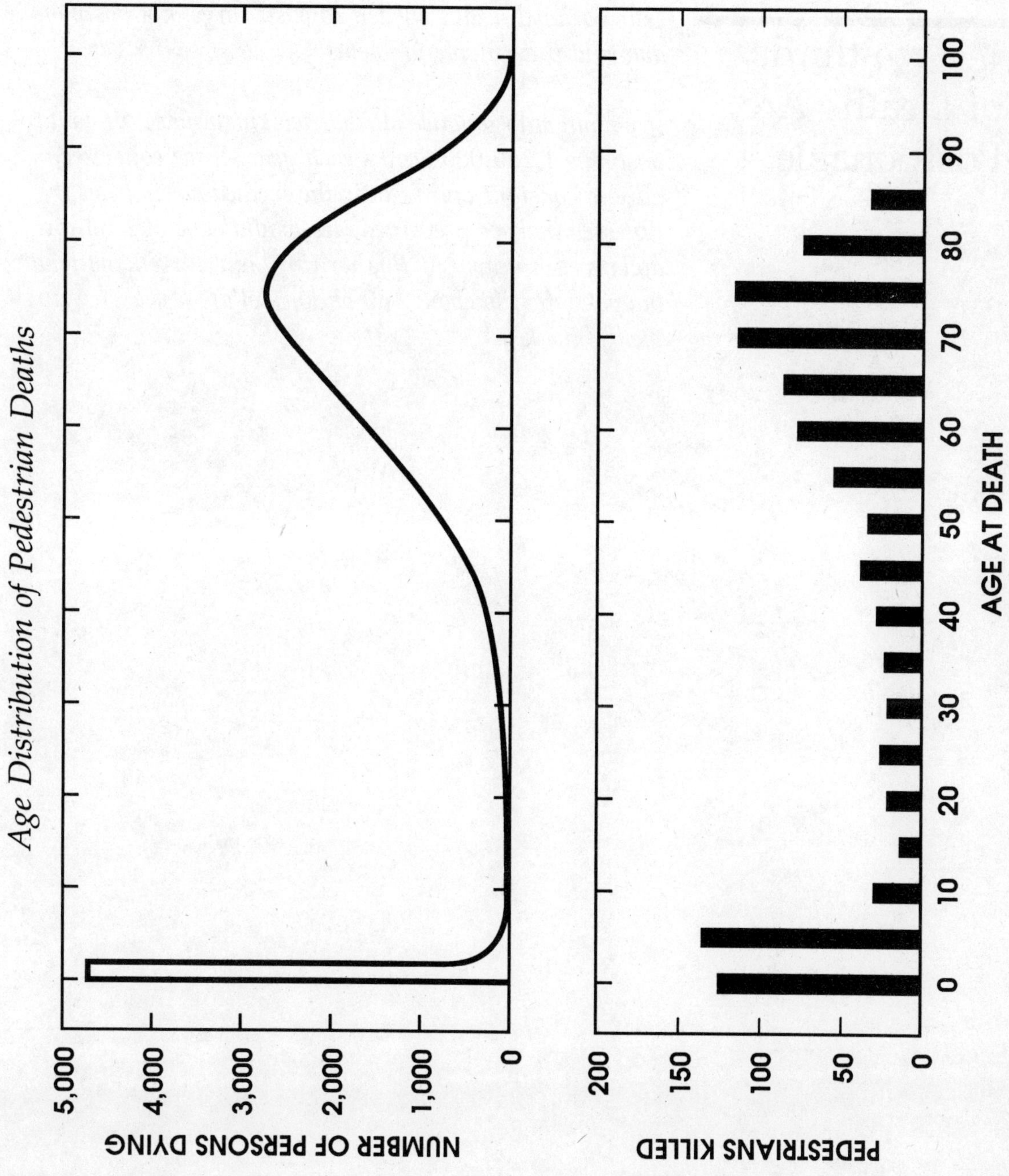

Age Distribution of Pedestrian Deaths
NUMBER OF PERSONS DYING
5,000
4,000
3,000
2,000
1,000
0
PEDESTRIANS KILLED
200
150
100
50
0
0
10
20
30
40
50
60
70
80
90
100
AGE AT DEATH

4/ Two-thirds of Deaths Are Postponable

Our national health burden consists largely of postponable and preventable problems.

If we put into practice all that we know now, we could postpone 1,260,000 deaths each year. If we could keep all else constant and recover the medical costs from the illnesses that we prevented, we would save 302 billion dollars each year. (At this writing, our current national budget deficit is about 160 billion dollars a year.) Aging well is the key.

Estimates of Potentially Postponable Deaths

Percent of Deaths Postponable	*Number of Deaths Postponable*	*Years of Life Lost Preventable*	*Economic Costs—$ Billions Preventable*
All—66%	**1,260,000**	**23,000,000**	**$302**
Injuries—90%	**144,000 (3)**	**5,490,000 (2)**	**75 (1)**
Circulatory disease—67%	**665,000 (1)**	**8,385,000 (1)**	**57 (2)**
Neoplasms—67%	**283,000 (2)**	**4,850,000 (3)**	**34 (3)**
Respiratory disease—76%	**98,000 (4)**	**1,359,000 (4)**	**25 (4)**
Digestive disease—55%	**41,000 (5)**	**779,000 (5)**	**23 (5)**
Musculoskeletal disease—30%	**1,700**	**32,700**	**6**
Infectious disease—50%	**38,000**	**708,000**	**5**

Rankings are shown in parentheses. From Tarlov, Kaiser Family Foundation, 1984.

5/ The Heart Disease Epidemic That Never Came

By 1960, heart disease had become the leading cause of death and was increasing rapidly. Experts (who always seem to be a bit alarmist) projected these increases into the future and wondered if the economy could stand all this disease.

In fact, smoking decreased, diets improved, and heart disease declined. Presently, the decline from heart disease has totalled over 40 percent in the last 20 years.

Moral: The future is not what we project, but what we make of it.

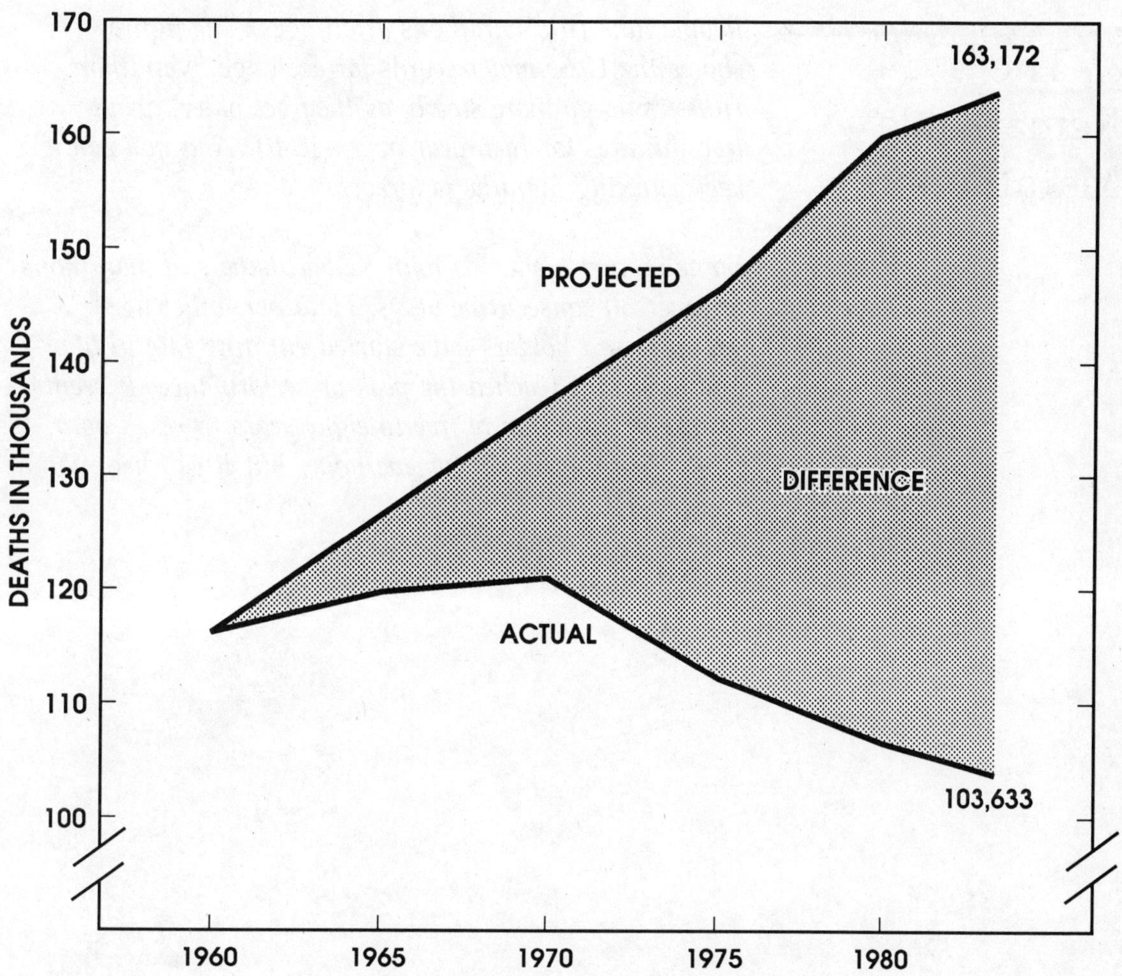

Deaths from Heart Disease for Persons 55–64 Years of Age and Projected Deaths: United States 1960–1982

Source: Division of Vital Statistics, National Vital Statistics System. Projections computed by Division of Epidemiology from data compiled by Division of Vital Statistics.

6/ The Remarkable Marathoners

People now run marathons at all ages. The figure shows the U.S. male records for each age. Marathon runners do go more slowly as they get older, about two minutes for each year over age 40. And you can't keep running marathons forever.

Some runners, such as John Kelley, have run marathons for over 50 consecutive years. However, other age-group record holders have started running late in life and have still reached the peak of performance. It seems to take a minimum of five to eight years to reach your peak. Running is not for everyone, but it can help you to age well.

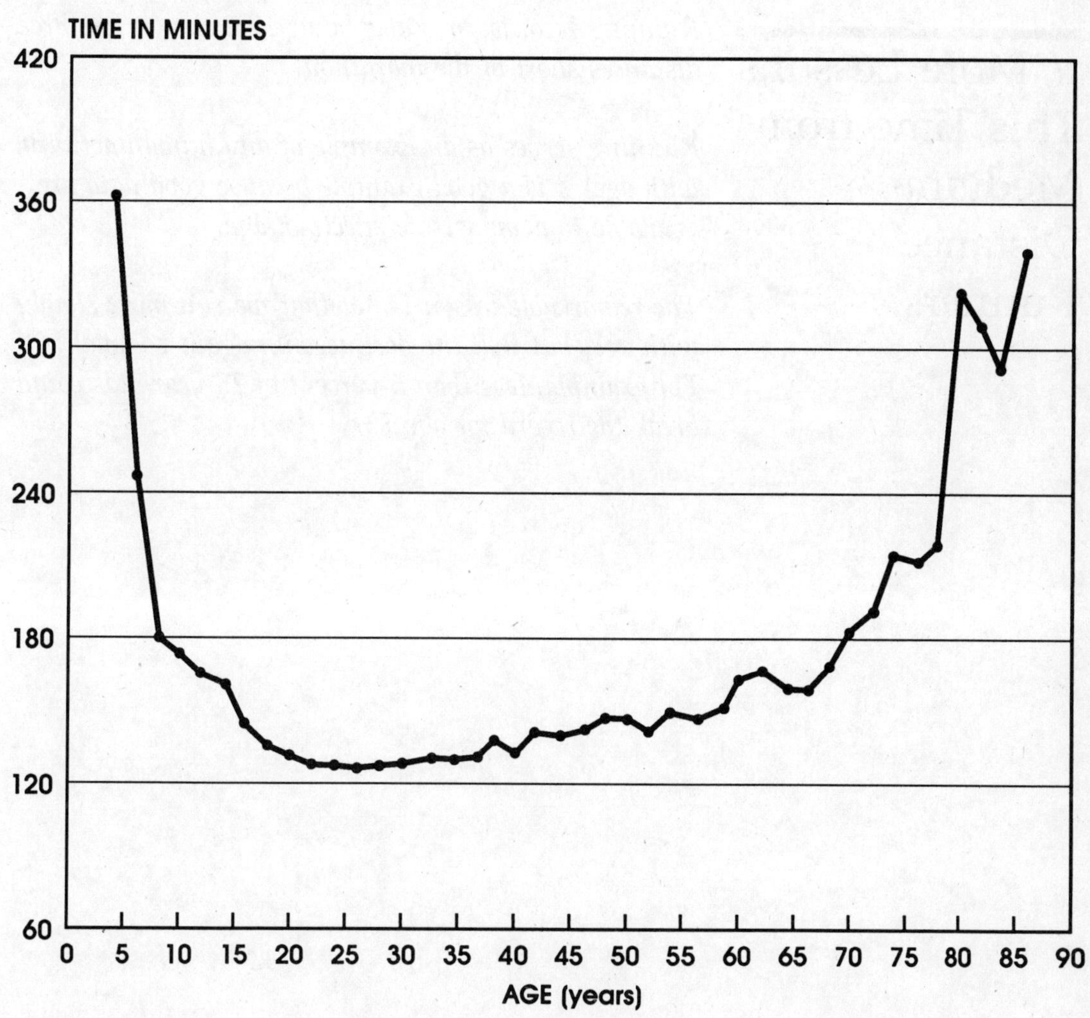

United States Marathon Age Records, 1986

7/ More Lessons This Time from Medium-Distance Runners

Running records for males by age are shown for three distances short of the marathon.

Running serves as an example of any human activity with age; it is a good example because good data are available to demonstrate effects of age.

The remarkable lesson is not that we run more slowly with age, but that the decline with age is so small! For example, less than 5 percent of 25-year-olds could break the record for age 75!

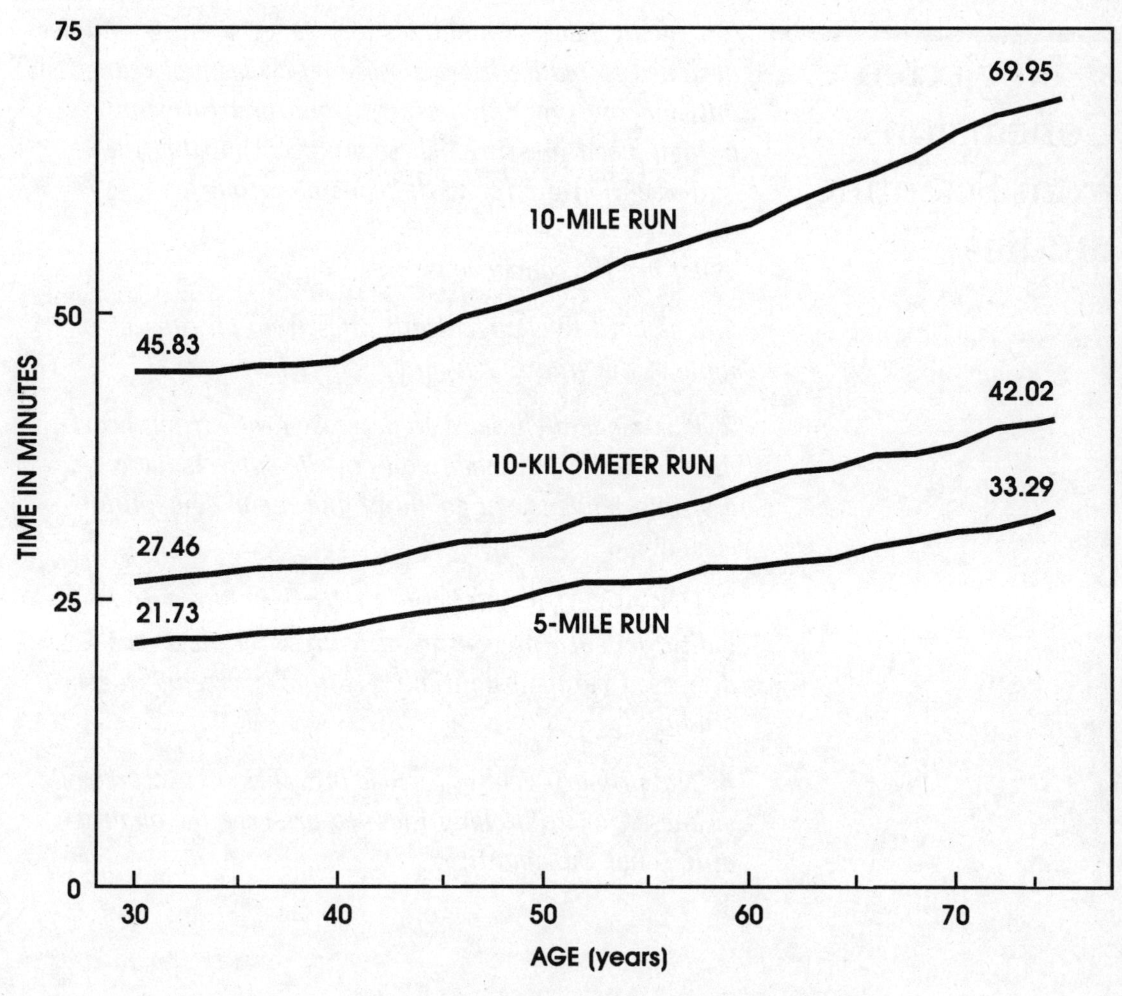

Running Records for Males

8/ Neglected Conclusions from Scientific Studies

The facing table summarizes four large scientific studies designed to reduce heart disease by cholesterol reduction, antismoking programs, aspirin, and/or treatment of high blood pressure. These studies compared the "intervention group" with "control" groups.

What are the conclusions?

1. *It is hard to change death rates from all causes; none of the studies had much effect here.*

2. *It is moderately hard to decrease deaths from heart disease itself, and when you do, the subjects have a strong tendency to go ahead and die of something else.*

3. *However, it is quite easy to decrease illness (morbidity) by such preventive measures. Sickness was decreased very substantially (16 to 37 percent) in every study.*

4. *The primary goal of disease prevention is to prevent sickness, not to prolong life—to preserve the quality of life, not the quantity.*

Major Randomized Trials of Primary Prevention

	Number of Men	Duration Years	DEATHS			CORONARY DEATHS			MORBID EVENTS			Morbidity Mortality
			Intervention	*Control*	*Diff/(%)*	*Intervention*	*Control*	*Diff/(%)*	*Intervention*	*Control*	*Diff/(%)*	
MRFIT[1]	**12,866**	**7**	**265**	**260**	**−5(−2)**	**115**	**124**	**9(7)**	**1,366**	**1,628**	**262(16.1)*****	**262/−5**
LRC[2]	**3,806**	**7**	**68**	**71**	**3(4)**	**44**	**32**	**12(27)**	**906**	**1,112**	**206(18.5)*****	**206/3**
Physicians[3]	**22,071**	**5**	**110**	**115**	**5(4)**	**5**	**18**	**13(72)****	**173**	**239**	**66(28)****	**66/5**
Helsinki[4]	**4,081**	**5**	**45**	**42**	**−3(−7)**	**14**	**19**	**5(26)**	**45**	**71**	**26(37)***	**26/−3**

*−p < .05, **−p < .01, ***−p < .001

[1]Morbid events: angina pectoris, intermittent claudication, congestive heart failure, peripheral vascular disease, stroke, accelerated hypertension, left ventricular hypertrophy, impaired renal function, total nonfatal coronary events.

[2]Morbid events: definite or suspect nonfatal coronary, positive exercise test, angina, coronary bypass surgery, congestive heart failure, intraoperative myocardial infarction, resuscitated coronary collapse, TIA, brain infarct, intermittent claudication.

[3]Morbid events: nonfatal coronary, nonfatal stroke.

[4]Morbid events: nonfatal coronary.

Sources: Multiple Risk Factor Intervention Trial Research Group, Coronary heart disease death, nonfatal acute myocardial infarction and other clinical outcomes in the multiple risk factor intervention trial, *Am J Cardiol* 1986;58:1–13; Lipid Research Clinic, Lipid Research Clinic coronary primary prevention trial results (1984), I, Reduction of incidence of coronary heart disease, *JAMA* 1984;251:351–364; The Steering Committee of Physicians' Health Study Research Group, Preliminary Report:Findings from the Aspirin Component of the Ongoing Physician's Health Study, *N Engl J Med* 1988;381:262–264; and M.H. Frick, O. Elo, K. Haapa, O.P. Heinonen, et al., Helsinki Heart Study: Primary-Prevention Trial with Gemfibrozil in Middle-Aged Men with Dyslipidemia, *N Engl J Med* 1987;316:1237–1245.

9/ Things Are Getting Better

Positive health changes do occur and are occurring. These changes are continuing, with improvement approximating 40 percent in most categories. Health benefits have occurred. More health benefits will occur in the future.

*Change in Per Capita Consumption of Various Products, 1963 to 1980**

Product	*Percent Change*
Cigarette tobacco	**−27.1**
Fluid milk and cream	**−24.1**
Butter	**−33.3**
Eggs	**−12.3**
Animal fats and oils	**−38.8**
Vegetable fats and oils	**+57.6**
Fish	**+22.6**

*Figures for calculating percentage changes obtained from the U.S. Department of Agriculture.

10/ Medical Costs Don't Necessarily Rise with Age

The two top lines in the facing figure show the increase in Medicare payments with age as popularly reported. Projections based on these data suggest very costly care for our future older population.

The flatter lines are the same data after costs for the individuals who died each year are taken out of the calculation. Medicare costs for those who survive a given year do not *increase with age. It is the high cost of death and the increase in the fraction of each successive age group who die that cause the apparent increase in costs per year. These high cost deaths are often painful, undignified, agonizing, and include a lot of intensive technical life support.*

Conclusion? If we can decrease the high cost of death we can greatly decrease high medical costs in older age groups.

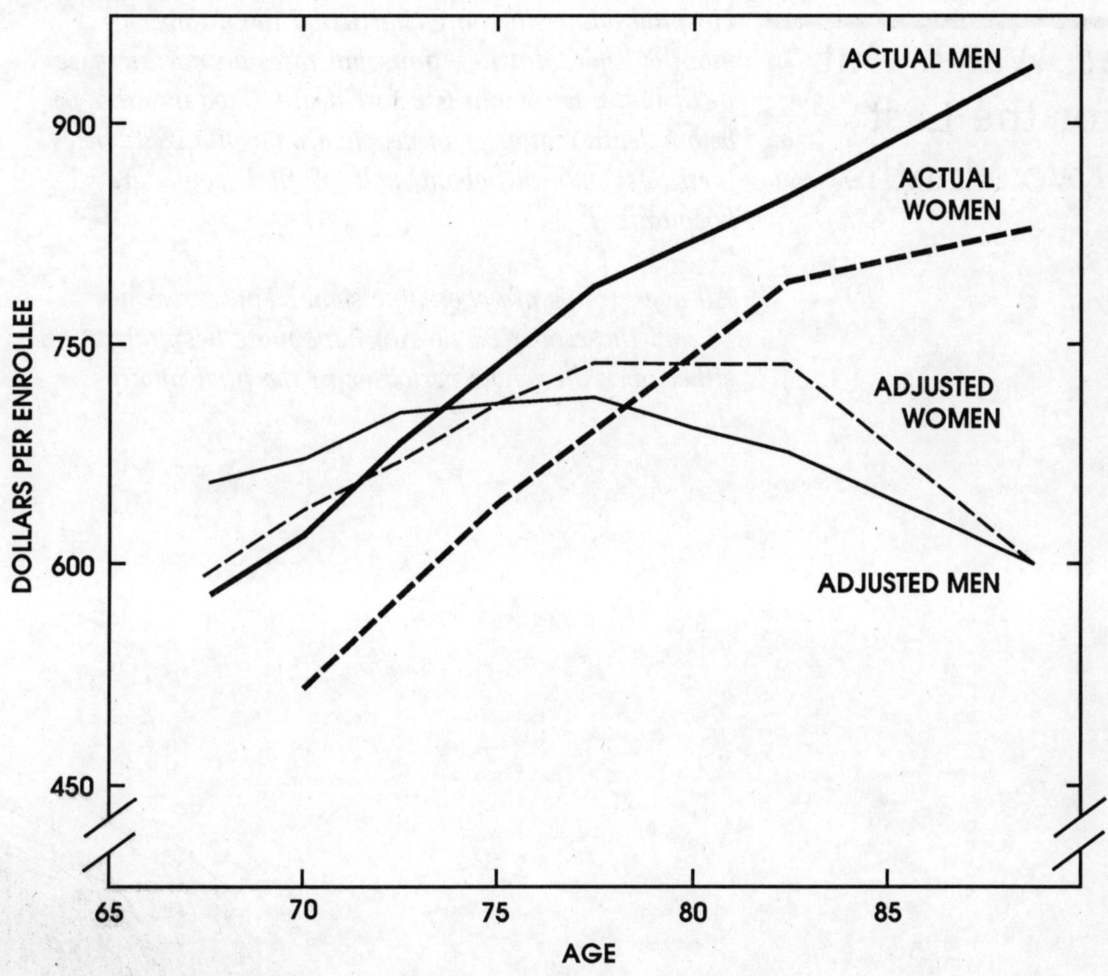

Medicare Reimbursement per Enrollee, Actual and Adjusted for Survival Status, 1976

11/ Watch Out for the Last Two Months

Hospital admissions are charted by the number of months before death. Admission rates do not increase until just a few months before death. Two months before death a quarter of people are hospitalized. In their last month, about half of the people are hospitalized.

All age groups are about the same. Those over age 75 and those over 85 do not *have more hospitalizations either over the whole period or in the final months.*

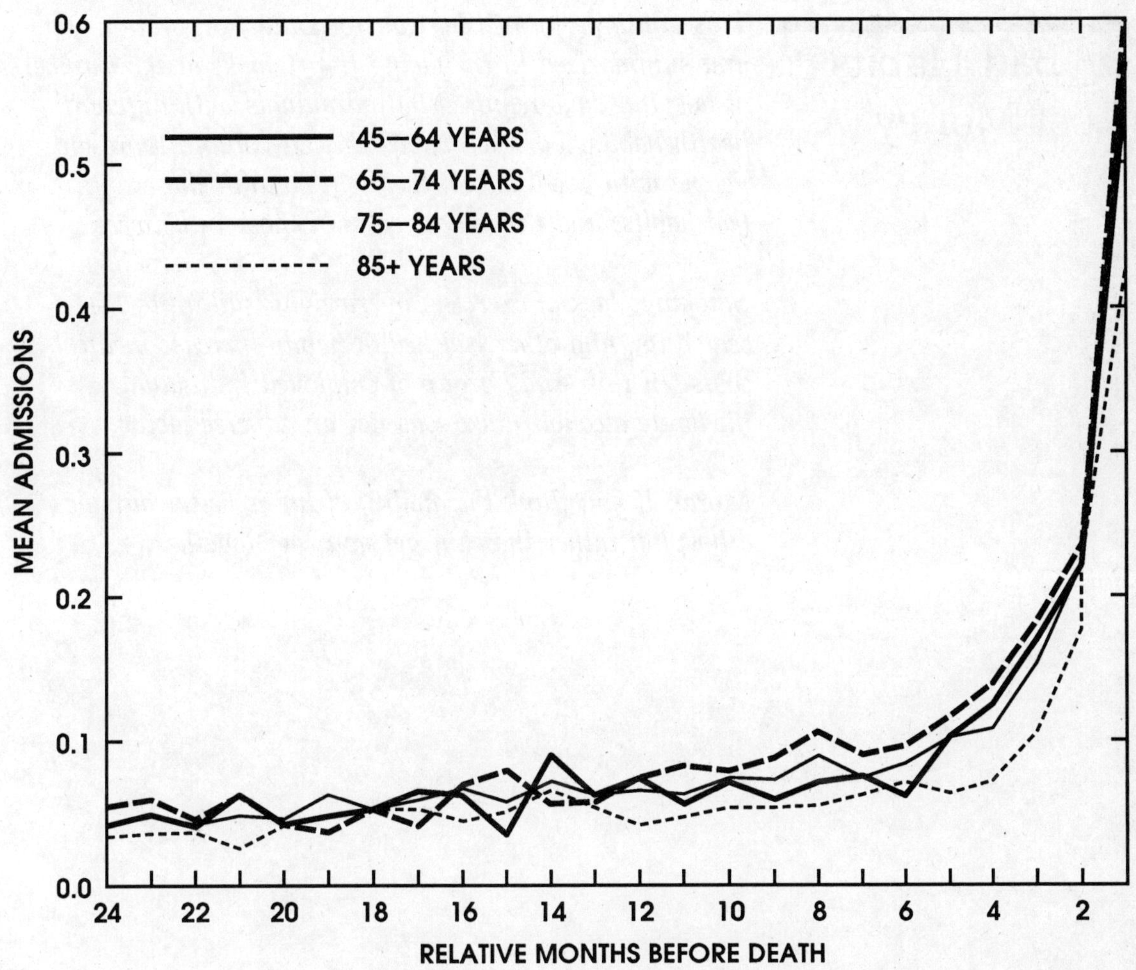

Hospital Admissions in the 24 Months Before Death

Source: Manitoba Health Services, 1976 (Roos and Montgomery).

12/ Bad Habits Cost Money

This study performed by Control Data Corporation and summarized in the facing figure looks at the number of hospital days required by individuals with different health habits. For each habit, the left column represents people with good habits, the right column those with bad habits, and the middle column those in between.

Smoking, lack of exercise, overweight, failure to use seat belts, and other bad health habits increase medical costs. In this study group of employed individuals, moderate alcohol intake was not an adverse factor.

Moral: If you think the quality of life is better outside a hospital rather than in, get your act together.

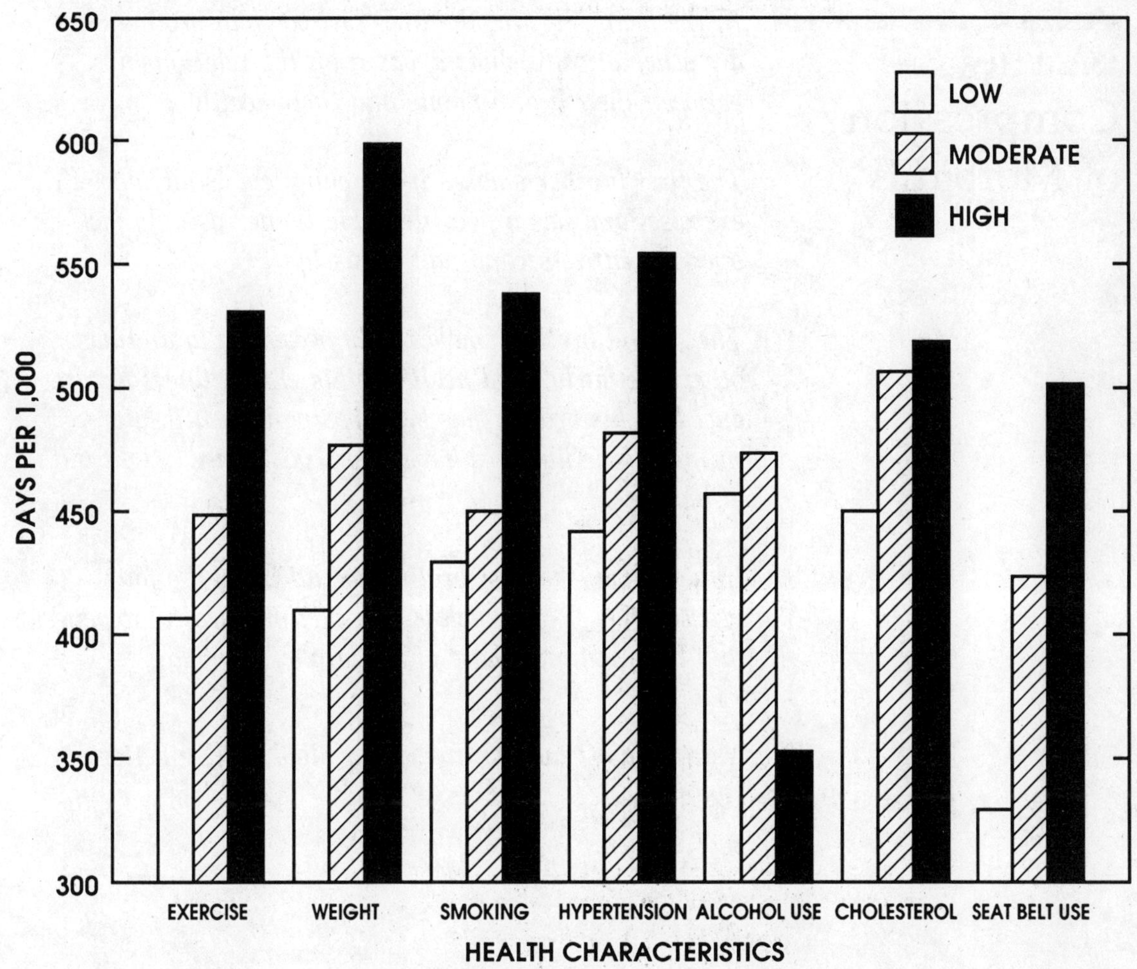

Hospital Inpatient Days per 1,000

13/ The Compression of Morbidity

In the facing figure, the lives of two twin brothers are schematically shown, based on the relationships between their health habits and their health.

The first brother smokes like a chimney, is fat, doesn't exercise, and has a poor diet. He is increasingly sick over the entire second half of his life.

The second brother smokes only occasionally and has otherwise fairly good health habits. Each illness experienced by his brother has been postponed until later in life. Some illnesses have been "postponed" right out of his life.

In actuality, the first brother would likely die four years earlier. Nevertheless, his lifetime medical expenses will be four times those of his brother.

Moral: Don't look to live longer, look to live better. Age well.

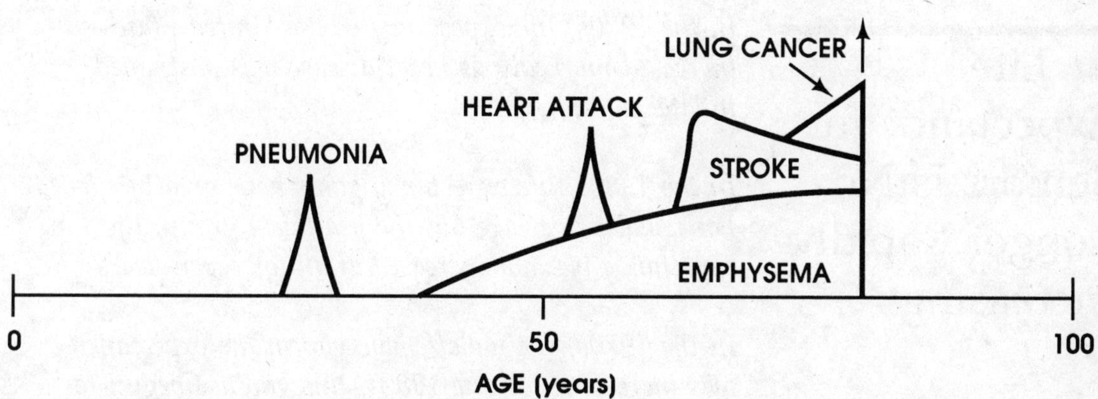

Prototypic Lingering Chronic Illness

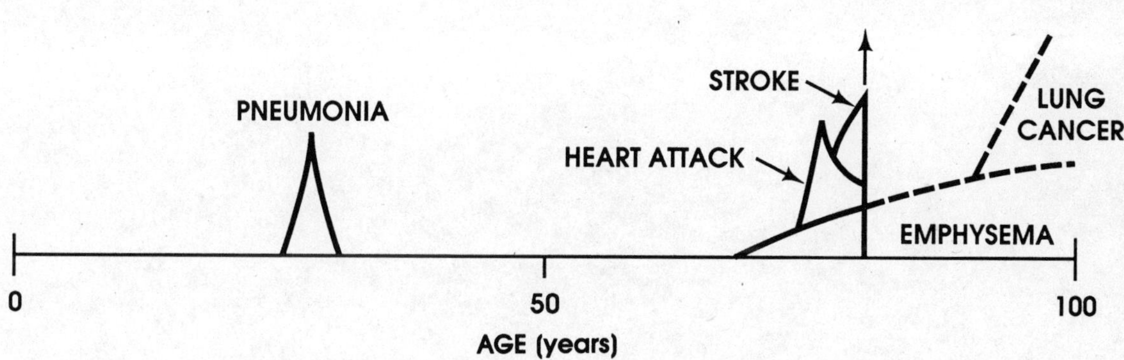

Effects of the Postponement of Chronic Disease

14/ Life Expectancy for Seniors Is No Longer Rapidly Increasing

In the 1970s, life expectancy in the United States increased markedly as heart disease was postponed to later ages.

In the 1980s, life expectancy gains have greatly slowed. For females over age 65, the healthiest group, life expectancy has not increased at all for seven years.

In the 1970s, the male/female gap in life expectancy was increasing. In the 1980s, this gap has begun to close. Males have been benefitting more than females from dietary changes, seat belt laws, and smoking cessation.

U.S. Changes in Life Expectancy, 1976–1986

From Birth	*1976*	*1977*	*1978*	*1979*	*1980*	*1981*	*1982*	*1983*	*1984*	*1985*	*1986*
All	**72.9**	**73.3**	**73.5**	**73.9**	**73.7**	**74.2**	**74.5**	**74.6**	**74.7**	**74.7**	**74.8**
Change	**.3**	**.4**	**.2**	**.4**	**−.2**	**.5**	**.3**	**.1**	**0**	**0**	**.1**
Males	**69.1**	**69.5**	**69.6**	**70.0**	**70.0**	**70.4**	**70.9**	**71.0**	**71.2**	**71.2**	**71.3**
Females	**76.8**	**77.2**	**77.3**	**77.8**	**77.4**	**77.8**	**78.1**	**78.1**	**78.2**	**78.2**	**78.3**
Male/Female Gap	**7.7**	**7.7**	**7.7**	**7.8**	**7.4**	**7.4**	**7.2**	**7.1**	**7.0**	**7.0**	**7.0**
From Age 65											
All	**16.1**	**16.4**	**16.4**	**16.7**	**16.4**	**16.7**	**16.8**	**16.7**	**16.8**	**16.8**	**16.9**
Change	**.5**	**.3**	**0**	**.3**	**−.3**	**.3**	**.1**	**−.1**	**.1**	**0**	**.1**
Males	**13.7**	**13.9**	**14.0**	**14.2**	**14.1**	**14.3**	**14.5**	**14.5**	**14.6**	**14.6**	**14.8**
Females	**18.1**	**18.3**	**18.3**	**18.6**	**18.4**	**18.6**	**18.7**	**18.6**	**18.6**	**18.6**	**18.6**
Male/Female Gap	**4.4**	**4.4**	**4.3**	**4.4**	**4.3**	**4.3**	**4.2**	**4.1**	**4.0**	**4.0**	**3.8**

Sources: Health, United States, 1986 DHHS Pub. No. (PHS)87-1232; Statistical Bulletin, Metropolitan Life Vol. 68, pp 8–14, 1987; Statistical Bulletin, Metropolitan Life Vol. 67, pp 18–23, 1988; Monthly Vital Statistics Report, Vol. 35, #13, Aug 1987. National Center for Health Statistics.

15/ Will the Experts Be Wrong—Again?

Experts tend to project past trends into future predictions. Because of the rapid rises of life expectancy in the 1970s, they projected similar increases in the future. As a result of neglecting the biology of aging, they used an assumption that increases will go on forever. But trees do not grow to heaven.

The 1982 Social Security projections are already seriously wrong with regard to female mortality. The 1987 middle-range projections also appear unlikely.

My bet? That we will remain at or below the 1987 low-range *Social Security projections through 1994.*

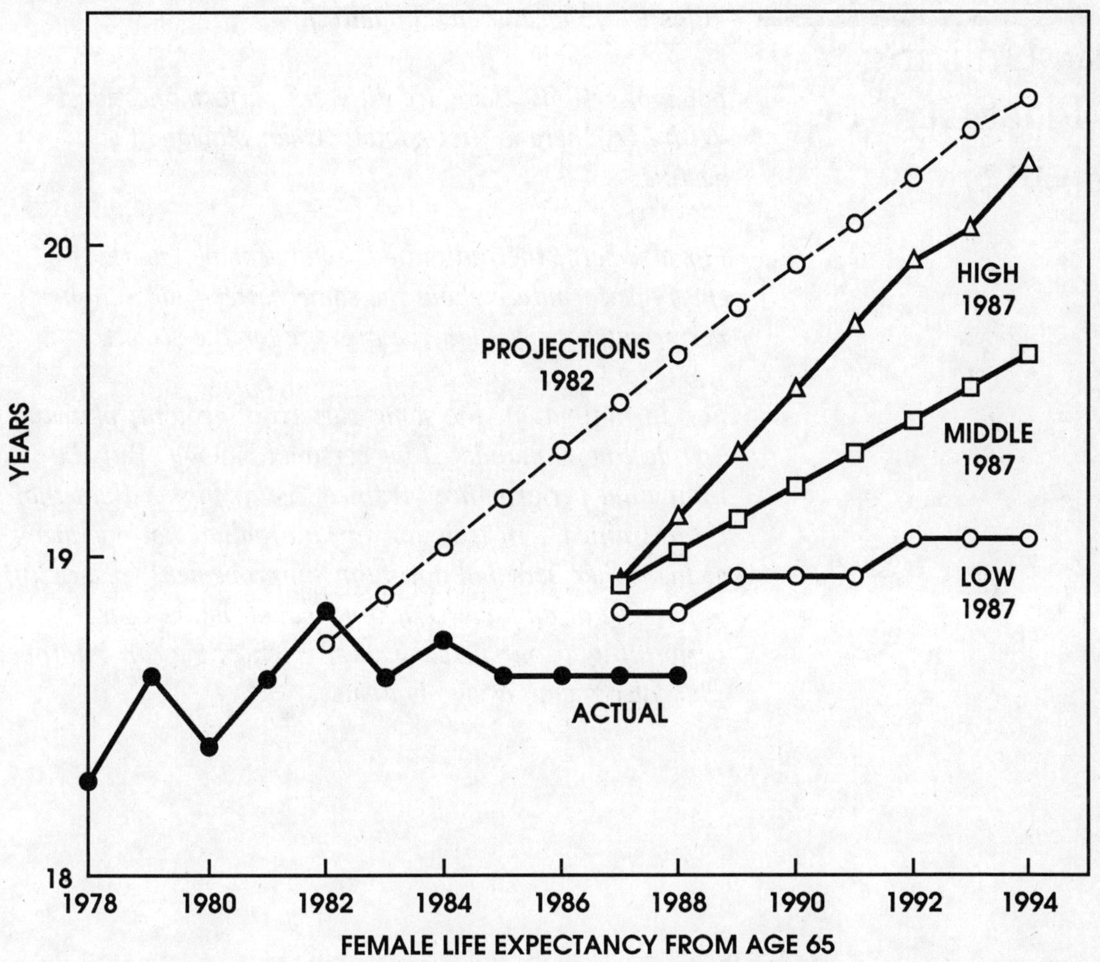

Social Security Projections and Actual Values, 1978–1994

Sources: Statistical Bulletin, Metropolitan Life Vol. 68 pp. 18–23, 1988; Social Security Area Population Projections, 1987; Actuarial Study No. 99, SSA Pub. No. 11–11546; Actuarial Study No. 87, SSA Pub. No. 11–11534, 1982.

16/ Utilizing "Plasticity" of Aging

"Plasticity" means "modifiability."

For any activity there are different performance levels. With age, there is first growth, then plateau, then decline.

For a society, the individuals who achieve "world class" performance show the same pattern, at a higher performance level than the average for the society.

For an individual, the same pattern of growth, plateau, and decline is mandated by personal biology. But the individual performance "trained" is far higher than that if "untrained." In fact, for any individual not operating at his or her personal optimum, improvement (plasticity) is possible at any age. Luckily, few of us are ever performing at our personal best. Hence, we can improve. The chief enemy of age is disuse.

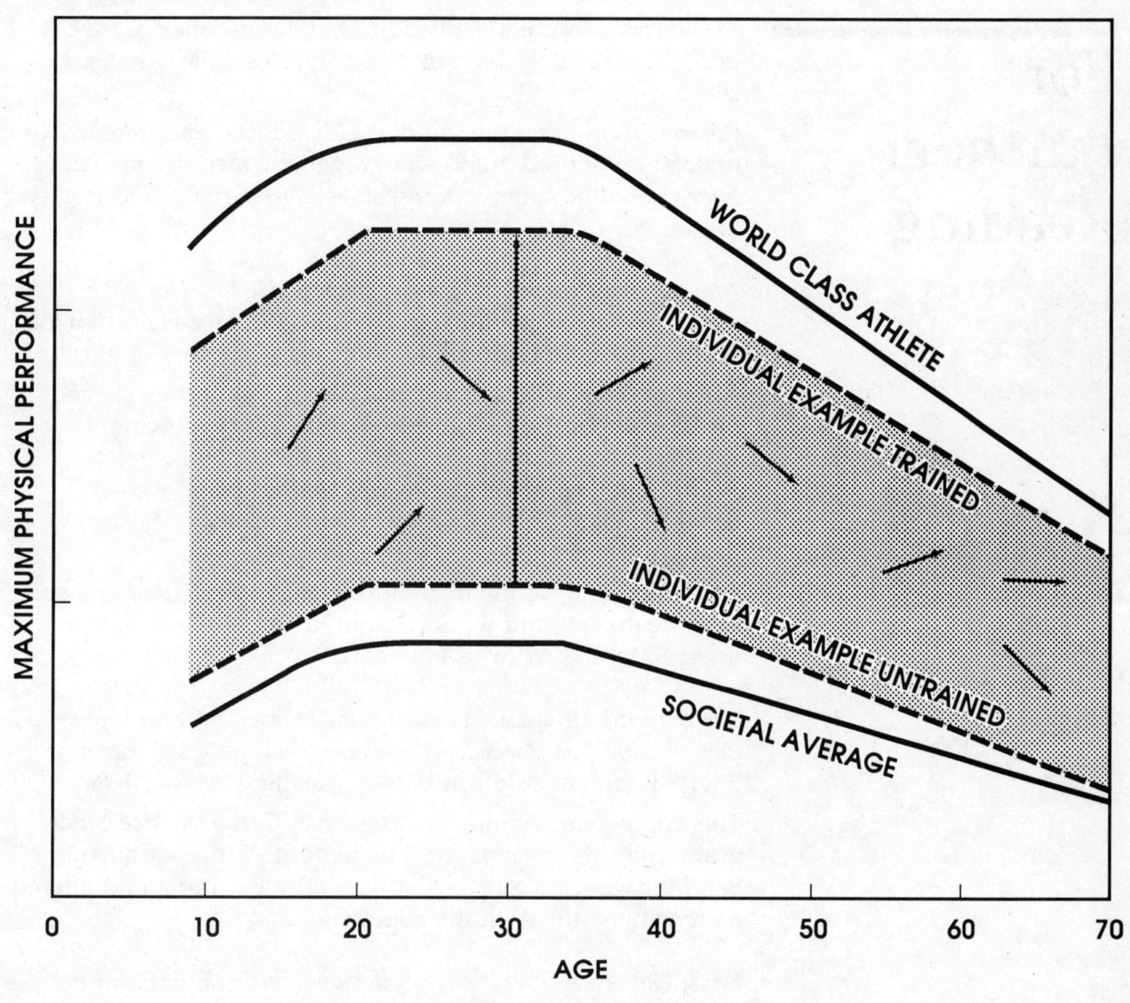

Patterns of Performance Levels

For Further Reading

About Your Medicines. United States Pharmacopeia Convention, Inc., 12601 Twinbrook Parkway, Rockville, Maryland 20852.

Reference on uses, precautions, side effects, and interactions of commonly used brand names, generic medications, and over-the-counter medications. Uses lay language and is easy to use.

An Ounce of Prevention: The Canadian Guide to a Healthy and Successful Retirement. Michael Gordon. Prentice-Hall, Canada, Scarborough, Ontario, 1984.

Another delightful and readable discussion of lifestyle and disease, duplicating other information yet reinforcing it.

Arthritis: A Comprehensive Guide to Understanding Your Arthritis. James F. Fries. Revised edition. Addison-Wesley, Reading, Mass., 1986.

Full description of the many forms of arthritis, their course, their treatment, and what you can do about them. Recommended by the Arthritis Foundation.

The Arthritis Helpbook: A Tested Self-Management Program for Coping with Your Arthritis. Kate Lorig and James F. Fries. Revised edition. Addison-Wesley, Reading, Mass., 1986.

This companion volume to *Arthritis: A Comprehensive Guide* grew from the syllabus for the Stanford Arthritis Center Self-Management courses developed by Dr. Lorig and offered nationally by the Arthritis Foundation.

Enjoy Old Age: A Program of Self-Management. B.F. Skinner and M.E. Vaughan. Norton, New York, 1983.

A personal account, extraordinarily insightful, from Dr. Skinner at age 79.

Fitness and Aging. John Piscopo. Wiley, New York, 1985.

An understandable if sometimes dry review of the principles and practice of exercise in older populations. Written for upper-division undergraduate and introductory graduate courses.

Growing Older, Getting Better: A Handbook for Women in the Second Half of Life. Jane Porcino. Addison-Wesley, Reading, Mass., 1983.

Feminine perspectives on aging past age 40, with good lists and references.

Growing Wiser. The Older Person's Guide to Mental Wellness. Donald W. Kemper, Molly Mettler, Jim Giuffre, Betty Matzek. Second edition. Healthwise, Boise, Idaho, 1988.

Fresh, varied, positive guide and workbook for seniors. Sound and often fun to read.

Handbook of Applied Gerontology. Gari Lesnoff-Caravaglia. Revised. Human Sciences Press, New York, 1987.

Multi-authored textbook written for health professionals but surprisingly lucid and readable. Has a very practical and positive perspective.

Home-Made Money: Consumer's Guide to Home Equity Conversion. American Association of Retired Persons, 1909 K Street, N.W., Washington, DC 20049, 1987. (free)

The best guide to reverse mortgages and similar transactions. AARP has other materials available as well.

Old Age Is Not for Sissies: Choices for Senior Americans. Art Linkletter. Viking Penguin, New York, 1988.

Another personal account, sprinkled with name-dropping, but surprisingly rich in practical perspectives on non–health-related issues.

Old Enough to Feel Better: A Medical Guide for Seniors. Michael Gordon. Fleet Books, Toronto, 1981.

A very readable and sound description of specific medical problems of seniors and their management. Can serve well to complement the discussions of this book.

The Power of Attorney Book. Denis Clifford. Second edition. Nolo Press, 950 Parker Street, Berkeley, Calif., 1988.

A guide through the complex legal environment of advance directives. Information about different state laws, different options available. Seventeen tear-out forms included for your use.

Take Care of Yourself. Donald M. Vickery and James F. Fries. Fourth edition. Addison-Wesley, Reading, Mass. 1989

The classic consumer's guide to medical care; the 5-million-copy best-seller that was the conceptual precursor of this book.

The 36-Hour Day: A Family Guide to Caring for Persons with Alzheimer's Disease, Related Dementing Illnesses, and Memory Loss in Later Life. Nancy L. Mace and Peter V. Rabins. Johns Hopkins University Press, Baltimore, Md., 1981.

This is a brilliant book on a nearly impossible subject. Written with sensitivity and understanding, it presents a realistic approach for the family or care giver of the demented patient.

Vitality and Aging. James F. Fries and Lawrence M. Crapo. Freeman, New York, 1981.

The scientific basis for human aging. The biologic and human factors that express growth and senescence. Full discussion of the compression of morbidity.

Wellness and Health Promotion for the Elderly. Ken Dychtwald. Revised. Aspen Systems, Rockville, Md., 1980.

Like all multi-authored books, content is uneven. Still, there is a lot of good information here, even if it doesn't all quite come together.

Many contributors to the literature of these issues have been omitted in this list of recommended readings. Some omissions have been deliberate. Note the total absence of any of the "*Fountain of Youth*" books that promise extreme longevity (less frequently good health) in return for taking some tonic (such as Vitamin C, Vitamin E, transcendental meditation, starvation, cold storage). Other omissions have been accidental; I will attempt to rectify serious omissions in future editions.

Index